I Second that
Emotion

Be Encouraged.
The Lord is your hope;
He will help you make it.

Pastor Dan...

I Second that *Emotion*

Unmasking the Seven
Plagues that Plague
Pulpits, Pews, and
Everyday People
Around the World

Darron L. Edwards

Foreword by Emanuel Cleaver, II
Former Mayor of Kansas City, Missouri

Pleasant Word

Packaged by Pleasant Word, PO Box 428, Enumclaw, WA 98022. The views expressed or implied in this work do not necessarily reflect those of Pleasant Word. The author(s) is ultimately responsible for the design, content and editorial accuracy of this work.

Unless otherwise noted, all Scriptures are taken from the Holy Bible, New International Version, Copyright © 1973, 1978, 1984 by the International Bible Society. Used by permission of Zondervan Publishing House. The "NIV" and "New International Version" trademarks are registered in the United States Patent and Trademark Office by International Bible Society.

Scripture references marked KJV are taken from the King James Version of the Bible.

Scripture references marked NASB are taken from the New American Standard Bible, © 1960, 1963, 1968, 1971, 1972, 1973, 1975, 1977 by The Lockman Foundation. Used by permission.

ISBN 1-4141-0310-7
Library of Congress Catalog Card Number: 2004097741

Dedication

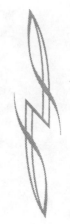

To my wonderful wife, supportive spouse, and best buddy, Michelle—You are always pushing me towards greatness. Thank you for showing me agape love! It is not what you say; it is really, what you do.

(First Corinthians 13: 4–7)

To my family—especially my mother and father, Don and Florence Edwards of Waxahachie, Texas, who reminded me when "smiles turned into snarls" to be faithful unto death and God will grant unto me the crown of life.

(James 1:12 and Revelation 2:10)

To my charming children—Darron, Jr., DeMarcus, Keianna, and Adrianna each of you have shown me that God has honored me by placing each of you in my life.

(Psalm 127:3)

To the amazing and supportive saints of United Believers Community Church, "A Place To Believe and Belong" in South Kansas City, Missouri—*www.believeandbelong.org*—thanks for the needed break and support to write this book.

Without a doubt, great things are in store for us. Thank you for believing in me!

(First Corinthians 11:1)

To all of the ministers and editors who honored me beyond measure by reviewing the manuscript during its development and then offering their comments as mentioned herein. Your technical guidance and support has made this work possible.

(Saint Mark 5:20)

You give me the inspiration and motivation to be transparent within this book,

I Second That Emotion

Table of Contents

Foreword

THE SEVEN CHAPTERS of this work are marked with maximum simplicity, sincerity, and seriousness. Preacher/writer Darron Edwards confronts, in this book, the knotty problems of anger, depression, grief, guilt, loneliness, stress, and quitting with the unquestionable confidence of the unflappable and inspired word of God.

The purpose of *I Second That Emotion* is to bless and build up. The language is profound but plain and the style is contemporary without being flashy.

Because human creatures are essentially what they think, those who furnish us with lofty thoughts are our most precious philanthropists. To be sure, this book is an act of noble giving. Additionally, this gift of thoughts on serious subjects will help those who preach, teach, and reach to do their job better.

There are seeds of salvation saturating this book. We are wise to plant them in the rich recesses of our mind where they find fertile and fair environs to flourish into spiritually nutritious fruitage.

—Emanuel Cleaver, II

Pastor, Saint James United Methodist Church of Kansas City, Missouri

Former Mayor of Kansas City, Missouri

Democratic Candidate (2004), United States Congress, Missouri (Fifth District)

Introduction

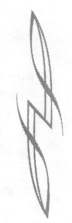

THIS BOOK IS for the everyday person. This practical application guide will inspire and motivate the individual who is
ready to tackle real life problems with real answers. God has
ordained that we live an abundant life filled with purpose and
possibilities in our wedded life, work life and worship life. This
book will expose the *seven plagues* that plague pulpits, pews,
and everyday people. Each emotion is explained with biblical,
textual, and transparent concepts that reach the heart and human soul.

How did I become a published author and writer? First, I
believe that it was a prenatal calling from God. However, I
acknowledged the gift much later in life. I believe that God
allows us to go through shades of darkness and despair so that
we can fully appreciate the wealth of His glory. After years of
successes and struggles, God was building within me the pages
of this discipleship study. I believe the gift of writing was birthed
in 1999 when I received the honor and grand opportunity to
preach at the prestigious Brookhollow Baptist Church in
Houston, Texas. This church, The Church Without Walls in
Houston, Texas, is a mega church of 16,000 plus members led

by Dr. Ralph Douglas West. On the morning of the conference, I became very ill. I thought that I might have to cancel my preaching assignment. However due to his meticulous selection of preachers, it was an honor to be invited. Therefore, I decided to preach in the event. After completing the message, I slumped in my chair. I was waiting on Pastor West to say to me that you preached a dynamic message. Instead, he looked me in my eyes and his first statement to me was, "You have a great gift of writing!" I am so grateful for that prophetic proclamation that pushed me to publish! Throughout my life, I have always known that my best expression comes through writing. As we endeavor to live a Christian life, I am convinced that the proverbial phrase of "life by the yard is hard and by the inch is a cinch" is a true statement. This book will help you move through life steadily as you encounter the many thrills and chills of the journey. Without a doubt, everything that you will read herein—*I Second That Emotion*!

Anger

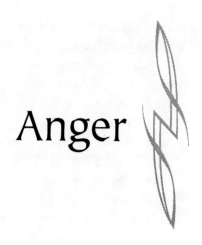

Scriptural Spotlight: Ephesians 4:26–27

"Be ye angry, and sin not: let not the sun go down upon your wrath:

Neither give place to the devil."

ANGER IS ONE **letter short of the word danger.** Like a wick on a stick of dynamite, anger is an emotion that is ready to explode. Learning to control our anger before our anger controls us is a life long learning experience. Anger is one of the most basic human emotions. Everyone gets angry. Anger is "an emotional state that varies in intensity from mild irritation to intense fury and rage," according to Charles Spielberger, PhD. Dr. Charles Spielberger is a psychologist who specializes in the study of anger. Anger is a feeling of antagonism. It is an emotion that sets people against each other. For example, recent surveys on marital violence report that approximately one in every seven American couples has used some form of physical abuse during an argument in the past year. Violence in arguments stems from a realization that we are not getting what we want when we want it. Like an infant who is feeling the hunger pangs of an empty tummy and demanding to have it satisfied with food, we too feel the pain of disappointed desires by expressing anger.

Unless we learn strategies to help us deal with our anger, our lives as well as others will be in constant danger. Growing up in Waxahachie, Texas, I can recall learning the following song: "If you are happy and you know it clap your hands, stomp your feet, and

> Anger shows up on your face

say Amen!" "If you are happy and you know it then your face will truly show it." This song teaches us that our internal state shows up in our external demeanor. In other words, whatever is troubling us on the INSIDE has a way of showing up on the OUTSIDE. In the words of the old Rhythm &Blues hit, "It's written all over your face, you do not have to say a word." As it relates to anger, you do not have to say it, nor shout it—others see it.

Because anger is so common to the human experience, and because it is such a threat to relationships, it is not surprising that the *Bible* has much to say about the dangers, roots, and taming of anger. When life displays "Dr. Jekyll and Mr. Hyde" qualities, how do you handle it? Has life ever made you mad? One National Baptist Convention preacher once said that we live in a world that has gone mad. It seems that when things turn out BAD in our lives, we tend to get MAD about life. Has life, in your opinion, turned out BAD for you?

For example:

- The doctor brings bad news about your cholesterol level despite a healthy diet.

- Your children bring home bad report cards despite countless tutors.
- Your employer brings a bad evaluation of your work performance despite your extra effort.
- Relatives bring up bad memories at the family reunion despite the improvements that you have made in your life.

When situations in life become seemingly out of control, we must not lose control. For example, it was reported by *Reuters*, reputed to be the world's largest international news agency, in Berlin that a furious German woman stormed out of the house armed with a hammer and smashed up a car. However, she vandalized the wrong vehicle. Only noticing the color, she had attacked her neighbor's blue Opel Corsa and not the blue Ford Fiesta belonging to her spouse.

Has anger ever distorted your view? What was the particular incident and how did you respond?

Yes, I immediately told on the person because I took it personally and am actual mare. My man did several things he shouldn't I thought - only after praying many days did I realize God is in control of what happens to me and when - not people. when I started to praying to fix myself, I felt I did better.

Has anger made you take out your vengeance on the wrong party? Please explain.

Don't recall that

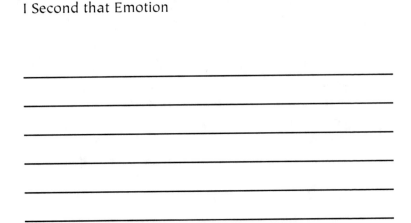

There are new terms that seek to expose our different anger types. One common expression is called road rage. **Road rage** is a term used to describe drivers who are disgruntled with the way others drive. Generally, these individuals take out their frustrations by blowing their car horns, by cutting into an individual's driving lane, or by making obscene gestures toward others. A perfect example of road rage happened when a man was rear-ended because he inadvertently pulled out in front of someone he should not have. Both drivers pulled to the side of the road to check the damage. The driver of the first car (driver A) took one look at his car and marched back to the second driver's car (driver B). Driver A immediately accused Driver B of causing the accident. An intense argument ensued and punches were thrown. Both Driver A and Driver B went to jail, not for the accident, but due to uncontrollable rage.

Air rage is a term used to describe disgruntled passengers who are growing increasingly upset with the airline industry. Thus, they take their frustrations out on airline personnel. For example, on an outbound flight from Tulsa to Dallas two men began to fight over an incident whereby one man

> We are now hearing new terms to describe uncontrollable anger.

leaned his seat back and seemingly invaded the space of the man sitting behind him. Not only did the two men fight each other but also attacked airline personnel who tried to resolve the conflict.

How does anger affect you? Anger can affect you in one of three ways. First, it can affect you **physically**. Anger can trigger physical problems that have been lying dormant such as hypertension, high blood pressure, heart, and stomach problems. Spielberger adds, "Like other emotions, anger is accompanied by physiological and biological changes. When you get angry, your heart rate and blood pressure go up, as do the levels of your energy hormones, adrenaline, and noradrenaline." Second, anger can affect you **emotionally**. When we are angry, it becomes difficult to make clear and accurate decisions. Finally, anger can affect you **spiritually**. Anger can disrupt your continuous fellowship with God and others.

Anger is a common emotion that all of us will experience in both positive and negative ways. In dealing with anger, you can either REPRESS IT, SUPRESS IT, or learn how to EXPRESS IT in a healthy and holy way.

ALTERNATIVE WAYS TO HANDLE ANGER

REPRESS IT

Repression is a form of denial. Repression happens when you decide to hold mental conversations in your mind about the occurrence without doing anything outwardly or verbally to handle it. For example, withholding sex (a repression tactic) often becomes a weapon of anger instead of the expression of shared love in a marriage. People who generally utilize the repression method usually focus more on the problem than the solution.

Do you believe that repression is a healthy alternative? Why or why not?

No- one day you're going to blow up over the smallest thing not even related to the depressed anger. Or you act out in ways you only end up hurting yourself rather than the person you intend to injure.

SUPPRESS IT

Suppression is the act of censoring or withdrawing. Because many people believe that anger is a sinful emotion, a common method used is to censor it. In our attempt to look like model Christians and citizens, we choose the suppression method in handling our anger. Most often, we end up pretending we are not angry in hopes that it will go away and no one will get hurt. After all, we reason, anger is not socially acceptable in church, home, or workplace. In suppressing anger, we are very much aware that we are angry, but for one reason or other, we choose to stifle expressing it and simply hold it inside of us. By doing this, we think we are neutralizing our feelings of anger, but actually we silently nurture it within and allow it to simmer on the back burner of our mind. Suppression can ultimately lead to bitterness, resentment, and unforgiveness.

Eventually when the suppressed anger is released, it is usually taking out on a less threatening, unsuspecting person. Often, that person is another family member.

Do you believe that suppression is a healthy alternative? Why or why not?

No - you end up resenting others, and you become bitter, angry bad moods homes will want to be around you which makes it worse for you.

EXPRESS IT

Expression is the communication of our beliefs and opinions. When you sense that anger feelings are emerging, ask yourself questions like these:

- Why do I feel angry?
- Where is my anger coming from?
- Why do I feel so threatened?
- Why is my anger so intense over something so small?

While we must learn to express our feelings, such expression must be done with discernment and regard for others. Those who express anger without love are "emotional dumpers." They back up their truckload of emotional garbage and unload it all over your front lawn. Naturally, we are born with the capacity to get angry and express the anger. A baby expresses anger by crying and yelling. However, as adults, we should not express our anger as babies do. Expressing your anger can be a productive procedure as long as it is released under control, corrective, and constructive, never destructive.

How have you expressed your anger in the past year?

Cried-yelled at my son and then
talked to him explaining what
I needed him to do & expected.

ADVANTAGES OF EARLY DETECTION

As a boy, I loved to eat my mother's tuna fish sandwiches. One particular day, I remember making my sandwich and seeing something green on my bread. I told my mother that something is wrong with this bread and she simply "pinched it off" and told me to eat it. I wanted another sandwich a few hours later; however, my mother detected a considerable amount of mole on the rest of the bread. My mother's early detection enabled me not to suffer the harmful effects of mole. It is the same principle as it relates to the subject of anger. Understanding how you react in the midst of threatening situations can help you overcome and deal with the harmful effects of anger.

One of the benefits of belonging to a *Bible* believing congregation is that you have the opportunity to fellowship with people who are going through the same perplexities of life that you are incurring. As it relates to this topic, anger is a hidden pain that comes to church every Sunday. Anger probably camps out in your house every day. Anger is also at your work place each workday. One of the great things about church worship is meeting people who will encourage you as you seek to live a life of productivity and promising potential. As it relates to anger, a healthy *Bible* based church can help you with early detection through relevant sermons and supportive small groups. What is a healthy church? A healthy church should not resemble a hospice. Hospices are places where people go to die. A church is a hospital. Hospitals are places where people take their pain with a hope and desire to get better. In essence, when they leave they want to leave better than they came. Likewise, church should be a haven for hurting people.

How often do you attend a place of public worship in a year? Do you feel good about the frequency of your attendance? If not, what will you do to change it?

Every Sunday - yes

Do you find attending corporate worship helpful? Why or why not?

Yes - I get encouragement & reminders of Gods promise, faithfulness & grace & mercy. It aint @ me.

_____

_____

_____

_____

_____

UNDERSTANDING THE DIFFERENT TYPES OF ANGER

HIDEOUS ANGER

In Ephesians 4:31, Paul uses the Greek word thumos. This word is translated **rage**. It literally describes a blazing fire or wildfire. This type of anger is sinful. What is sin? E. Paul Hovey defines sin as having four characteristics: "self-sufficiency instead of faith, self-will instead of submission, self-seeking instead of benevolence, and self-righteousness instead of humility." Hideous anger (rage) is a harmful and sinful anger that spreads like wildfire. Generally, it will consume everything in its path. According to the **Federal Emergency Management Agency (FEMA)**, WILDFIRES usually begin in DRY PLACES. Spiritually, rage erupts in the midst of dry places and people. Any place or person that only receives a SPRINKLE OF GOD'S LOVE or a DRIZZLE OF HIS FORGIVENESS is a potential WILDFIRE. Frankly, when there is no evidence of SPIRITUAL RAIN in your life, God does not REIGN over your life.

Ephesians 4:31 admonish us to "Let all bitterness, and wrath, and anger, and clamor, and evil speaking, be put away from you, with all malice." In other words, Apostle Paul helps us to realize that being involved in this type of anger could make us lose so much more than just our temper. You can lose your job, joy, and jeopardize your life or someone else's. This type of anger made Cain kill Abel, Saul lose his throne, and Moses smite the rock.

The following illustration from *The National Geographic*, November 1985, helps us to understand the harmful effects of anger. The article describes a national park ranger in British Columbia who owns two sets of huge antlers, as wide as a man's reach, locked together. The story goes that evidently two bull moose began fighting, their antlers locked, and they could not get free. They died due to anger. What pressing issue is going on in your life that makes you want to "lock horns" with someone and refuse to let go?

Have you experienced this type of stubborn anger? What happened?

> *yes but I didn't let it kill me completely. I prayed I asked God to help me let it go. To help me forgive forget & move past it*

HIDDEN ANGER

In contrast, Ephesians 4:26 says, "Be ye angry, and sin not: let not the sun go down upon your wrath." In this passage, Apostle Paul uses another Greek word for anger. PERORGISMO is the Greek word used to represent hidden anger.

Thumos anger, as described earlier, is rage expressed. Perorgismo anger, or hidden anger, is rage repressed.

Thumos anger is like an erupting volcano.

Perorgismo anger is like a smoldering volcano.

Perorgismo can become Thumos. Hidden anger can become hideous anger by simple agitation! Quite simply, agitation can make RAGE come out of its CAGE! A story is told of a young woman who met with her family deacon about her upcoming divorce. The young woman exclaimed, "I am mad that my husband left me. However, I am in rage that he left me broke."

What pressing problem in your life is beginning to make rage come out of its cage?

My son's disobedience of teen years

WHAT IS YOUR BOILING POINT?

Proverbs 14:17 says, "He that is soon angry dealeth foolishly and a man of wicked devices is hated." Another *Bible* translation of the same passage says, "A quick tempered man does foolish things." What does it take to make you blow your stack? Some people lose their temper over seemingly insignificant things. An old proverb says, "The emptier the pot, the quicker it boils." Chemistry teaches us that the less water in the pot; the quicker you reach a boiling point. WATER in certain *Bible* passages is a symbol of the Holy Spirit. In other words, the less the Holy

Spirit has of you, the quicker you act as if you do not have the Holy Spirit. Everyone has a boiling point, and the first step in dealing with anger is recognizing our personal boiling point. Science teaches us that the boiling point of water at sea level is 100 degrees. However, the higher the altitude the longer it takes water to boil. In short, the higher you are in God, the longer it takes you to boil. *focus on going higher*

HOLY OR HEALTHY ANGER

Not all anger is sinful. In Ephesians 4:26, Paul says, "Be ye angry, and sin not." Another *Bible* translation says, "In your anger do not sin." This is called holy anger or righteous indignation. Righteous indignation means that I have, as a Christian, a

> Healthy anger is based on the right grounds, against the right persons, in the right manner, at the right moment, and for the right length of time

RIGHT to be angry about things that make God angry. One definition of holy anger or righteous indignation is when an individual is angry on the right grounds, against the right persons, in the right manner, at the right moment, and for the right length of time. Once again, anger alone is not wrong! Only when you mix anger with something else does it become wrong!

- Cigarettes are strong but mixed with formaldehyde the effect becomes stronger.
- Alcohol is strong but mixed with drugs the effect becomes stronger.
- Anger is strong but mix it with jealousy, envy, and rage it becomes stronger.

Exhibiting holy anger, in my personal life, helps me to understand that HATE HURTS THE HATER MORE THAN

THE HATED. Galatians 5:20–24 states, "Now the works of the flesh are manifest, which are these; adultery, fornication, uncleanness, lasciviousness, idolatry, witchcraft, hatred, variance, emulations, wrath, strife, seditions, heresies, envyings, murders, drunkenness, revellings, and such like: of the which I tell you before, as I have also told you in time past, that they which do such things shall not inherit the kingdom of God. But the fruit of the Spirit is love, joy, peace, longsuffering, gentleness, goodness, faith, meekness, temperance: against such there is no law. And they that are Christ's have crucified the flesh with the affections and lusts."

As you examine your own life, how would you describe your fruit (maturity level)?

They are all present & operating in my life most of the time.

Moreover, if anger, selfishness, and envy are high on the list, this indicates that you need the work of the Holy Spirit to help you in your anger moments.

Anger, I have been there. I second that emotion!

SMALL GROUP DISCUSSION QUESTIONS:

1. List five instances that caused you to become angry.

   unclean room - not doing work @ home
   bad grades   on phone
   talk back w/ body language

2. Write a short sentence prayer that expresses your angry feelings to God.

   Lord I feel like I do more than above to ask for my child yet he is
   ungrateful - help me to hand you a your child so we can become as new

3. What strategies did you employ to help deal with your anger? Do you believe that you utilized healthy strategies? If not, explain.

   Yelled, cat slide yelled. talked finally beat. Most of the time. Should have beat earlier.

4. Do you believe that the author's revelation of healthy or holy anger can help you in your anger moments? Why or why not?

   yes - know that some he + get out of hand

5. Do you agree that hate hurts the hater more than the hated? Why or why not?

   yes because for the most part our hate is focused on things not of god - thus it comes from Satan

27

Depression

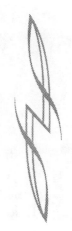

Scriptural Spotlight: Psalm 42:3

"My tears have been my meat day and night, while they continually say unto me, Where is thy God?"

WHAT IS DEPRESSION? Depression is not just sad-ness; it is a state of mind that makes it difficult for people to envision that any activity they engage in will turn out well. A man asked a preacher friend, "How many active members do you have?" The preacher replied, "They are all active." He continues his comment by expressing, "Half of them are working with me, and half of them are working against me." Sometimes in life, we find that some people are working against us rather than for us. This can bring on depressing thoughts. The book, *Silent Pain,* draws upon several considerations as it relates to depression in order that we might perform our own personal evaluation:

- Do you feel consistently sad or numb nearly every day?
- Do you have little or no interest in activities that you used to find enjoyable?
- Do you have difficulty sleeping?

- Do you feel you are sleeping too much?
- Do you feel tired most of the time?
- Do you find it hard to concentrate or stay focused?
- Has your interest in marital intimacy lessened?
- Do you feel overwhelmed by the burdens of life?
- Do you think about death or killing yourself?

If you can identify with most of the above questions, chances are you are dealing with deep depression. Depression is a serious struggle, and there are usually no simple or quick solutions. Reading Psalm 42 will help you to discover that a depressed person feels like a helpless and hopeless individual. In fact, depression affects every core of your being. According to First Thessalonians 5:23, you are a body, a soul, and a spirit. When God created you, He made you with a body, a soul, and a spirit. Depression can cause physical problems (body), emotional problems (soul), spiritual problems (spirit), or a combination of any of these. One of England's finest preachers was an ordinary man by the name of Charles H. Spurgeon. Frequently during his ministry, he plunged into severe depression. In dealing with depression, the following words of Spurgeon hold true today. "There are dungeons beneath the castles of despair." This is a great definition of depression. Depression can mask itself in many other forms. According to the *Diagnostic and Statistical Manual of Mental Disorders (fourth ed.), American Psychiatric Association,* "depression can cause rapid weight loss, irritability, hypersomnia, or inappropriate guilt"; thus, depression really does create dungeons beyond the castles of despair.

Depression is expressed utilizing the following poem:

We, the Depressed, in our darkest hours have
No energy to move
No reason to live
No will to survive

No hope in a cure
No reason to try
We roam the earth as the living dead
Wanting only to extinguish
That persistent heart that beats,
That ceaseless breath that enters,
That pain that never relents
Every cell of our being wants to die,
Yet We Live!

—Anonymous

Are you able to identify with this poem? Please explain.

_____

_____

_____

_____

_____

_____

_____

Statistics vary on this subject; however, approximately eight million people in America are affected by depression. The **National Institute of Mental Health** discloses on their website "depression is one of the most common conditions associated with suicide in older adults. Depression is a widely under-recognized and under-treated medical illness. In fact, several studies have found that many older adults who die by suicide—up to 75 percent—have visited a primary care physician within a month of their suicide." Moreover, studies reveal that women are twice as likely to be treated for depression; however, men are four or five times more likely to commit suicide. This indicates that women more easily admit their depression and seek therapy for it, while men tend to be out of touch with their feelings of emptiness. Dr. Ivan Goldberg, a psychiatrist and clinical psychopharmacologist in private practice in New York City, shares a startling revelation that some depressed individuals are "treatment resistant." Is there any help for depressed individuals who do not respond to over the counter medications?

UNDERSTANDING DEPRESSION

Grief is not depression

It is important to recognize the differences between depression and other emotional problems. For instance, depression should not be confused with grief. When one experiences the loss of someone or something precious, that person passes through the process of grief. This grieving process is healthy and normal. Grief is not depression; however, if grief is not resolved it can deteriorate into long-term, dangerous depression.

Again, grief is not depression.

Guilt is not depression

Do not confuse depression with guilt. When a person sins or commits a shameful act, he experiences nagging guilt. This guilt is not depression, because a feeling of guilt is normal for sinful behavior. Our God-given conscience causes us to feel remorse and pain over sin. For a Christian, forgiveness from guilt can be found in Jesus Christ. When we confess our sins and repent our guilt is replaced with a sense of gratitude for God's forgiveness. Again, guilt is not depression.

Loneliness is not depression

Loneliness is a signal that something is missing in your life. Loneliness is a feeling of being unneeded, unloved, unwanted, and even unnecessary. It is a desperate sense of "Nobody needs me." "Nobody wants me." "Nobody loves me." Loneliness is not depression; however, if loneliness is not resolved—it can deteriorate into long-term, dangerous depression. Again, loneliness is not depression.

Gary Collins' well-researched work, *Christian Counseling*, identifies four basic types of depression:

Endogenous depression is caused by a chemical imbalance in the central nervous system. In addition, endogenous depression is a term used to describe patients who do not respond to medication.

Reactive depression is a response to severe personal disappointment. It may be caused by divorce, loss of job, or loss of health.

Toxic depression is caused by the influence of outside substances on the nervous system. Alcohol, drugs, diet, or a virus may lead to toxic depression. When the damaging substance is removed, the depression leaves.

Psychotic depression is caused by a combination of factors that often lead to a nervous breakdown or burnout. Psychotic depression combines depression with hallucinations or delusions.

Have you experienced any of these four basic types of depression? Please explain.

_____

_____

_____

_____

_____

_____

_____

IDENTIFYING THE CAUSES OF DEPRESSION

The following information shared from GlaxoSmithKline, a world leading research-based pharmaceutical company, helps us to become more aware of the causes of depression. "Some of the more common factors involved in depression are:

Family history - Genetics play an important part in depression. It can run in families for generations.

Trauma and stress - Things like financial problems, the breakup of a relationship, or the death of a loved one can bring on depression. You can become depressed after changes in your life, like starting a new job, graduating from school, or getting married.

Pessimistic personality - People who have low self-esteem and a negative outlook are at higher risk of becoming depressed. These traits may actually be caused by low-level depression, also called dysthymia.

Physical conditions - Serious medical conditions like heart disease, cancer, and HIV can contribute to depression, due to physical weakness and stress. Depression can make medical conditions worse, since it weakens the immune system and can make pain harder to bear. In some cases, depression can be caused by medications used to treat medical conditions.

Other psychological disorders - Anxiety disorders, eating disorders, schizophrenia, and (especially) substance abuse often appear along with depression."

As you identify potential causes of depression, which factors listed above could be affecting you? Please explain.

_____

_____

_____

_____

_____

_____

Most times, people express the desire to be like *Bible* characters because they believe that *Bible* characters were free from pain and difficulties. Nothing could be further from the truth.

> Enough is Enough

We can learn much about depression by studying the life of Elijah. First Kings 19:1–9, portrays Elijah sitting under a juniper tree praying these words of despair, *"It is enough; now, O LORD, take away my life."* Does that sound familiar? Have you ever confessed to God or anyone that you have had more than you can take?

Careful research into the life of the prophet Elijah reveals some of the causes of depression from a biblical perspective. First Kings 19 describes how we are most vulnerable to depression when we are **physically drained**. When you become tired and run down, you are a prime candidate for depression. Elijah found himself in the depths of depression after he had been involved in a stressful confrontation on Mount Carmel. To explain this point a well-known pastor utilized the following illustration to define exasperation that can lead to depression. "Do you recall watching circus performances whereby a person spins plates on top of poles? He would spin a plate on top of a pole, run to the next pole, spin a plate on top of it, and then run and do the same with another. He would do this until all of the plates were spinning at one time. Then he would run from pole to pole and spin the plates to keep them going." This illustration describes the life-style of many people. Many of us have so many plates spinning that our lives are spent running from one project to another, trying to maintain balance. When our bodies get tired, we are susceptible to depression.

Do you feel physically drained while carrying out your daily routine? Please explain.

_____

_____

_____

_____

_____

_____

Second, we are vulnerable to depression when we are **emotionally depleted**. Not only was Elijah physically tired, he was emotionally emptied. He had been dealing with difficult people. He was being threatened by Jezebel and her husband Ahab. If you are not careful, people will drain you emotionally.

There are times when all of us need to draw positive energy from those around us. When that does not occur, on a consistent basis or in moments of need, it can lead us into emotional turmoil. Elijah began to feel afraid, nervous, and desperate. Each of these emotions is indicative of how depression can make an individual feel.

Have you ever felt these emotions? What caused these feelings to surface?

_____

_____

_____

_____

_____

_____

_____

Third, we also get depressed when we are **spiritually defeated**. In addition to Elijah's physical and emotional problem, he suffered from a spiritual problem. After a great spiritual victory, Elijah felt like a loser. One of the signs of depression is a mood swing. Elijah began to delve into the area of self-pity. Self-pity is a spiritual problem. One of the strangest creatures ever created is the ostrich. An ostrich has a defense mechanism of hiding when trouble comes. The ostrich is a master in hiding from the realities that are all around. However, the ostrich only hides his head. The body of the ostrich is still exposed. Is the ostrich really hidden from others? When we are depressed, we must not develop an "ostrich mentality." Though we may hide out, it is quite apparent that something is drastically wrong. According to the **Center of International Education at the University of Massachusetts at Amherst**, "when you feel devalued, useless, and helpless—these feelings can dominate your life experiences." Perhaps these feelings invaded the prophet Elijah and that is why we find him at a dry brook under a juniper tree feeling depressed.

Can you recall an experience in which you felt spiritually defeated? Please explain.

_____

_____

_____

_____

_____

_____

_____

OVERCOMING DEPRESSION

Once again, positive people struggle with depression. The good news comes when you discover that there is hope in God. While in the valley of the shadows of despair, you can discover that Jesus is the Lily of the Valley. In Psalm 42:5, David identifies the key when he said, "**HOPE** thou in God."

What is Biblical hope?

- Biblical hope is trusting in the expectation of the revelation!
- Biblical hope believes that you will receive!

- Biblical hope is standing on the promise that what has *been* will not always *be!*

Having hope is as important as water is to fish and electricity to a light bulb.

- Without hope, students get discouraged and drop out of school.
- Without hope, athletic teams keep losing.
- Without hope, authors stop writing, inventors stop inventing, and artist stop drawing.
- Without hope, addicts return to their habits and churches stop praying.

Hope will put a smile on your face when life tries to make you frown.

Hope will keep you upbeat about life when others are feeling down.

Most certainly, hope will move you to act on faith when no one else believes.

I have broken HOPE down acrostically so that we might better understand this point and escape the depths of depression.

Honor the process and stick with it

In our "microwave society," people are always looking for a quick fix. They want a pill to take or a book to read that will immediately relieve their depression. One author wisely suggests, "If you are in a depressed state, think of yourself as a car battery that needs recharging. When a battery loses its charge, it may recharge two ways. A mechanic can put a **quick charge** into the battery or he can use the **trickle charge** method. A

> Allow God to recharge your life

quick charge will recharge the battery, but it may cause further damage of the battery. However, the trickle charge method gradually introduces a small amount of power until the battery is completely recharged." This is the most effective way to recharge a battery. In fact, it is perhaps the most efficient way to recharge a life. While most of us are looking for a quick charge, God wants to renew us through a slower, more stable process.

Open Up To God

Struggling people should not sit in silence. Far too many of us sing with our lives "I Surrender Some" instead of the well-known hymn "I Surrender All." One of the common areas that most people struggle in or fail to surrender is in the area of communicating with God and others. We must learn how to express our innermost feelings to God using honest, open, and transparent communication. Opening up to God helped to draw Elijah out of depression. When Elijah began to dialogue with God, our Heavenly Father rendered unto Elijah a miraculous illustration of how to hear from Him. God took Elijah to a mountain in Horeb. God then amazed Elijah with a divine demonstration of lightning, rain, thunder, and earthquakes. Elijah was looking for God, but he did not find Him in that dramatic and public demonstration. Instead, God spoke to him in a whisper. In this quiet time with God, Elijah was reassured that God was still in control. God understands that we are private people who like to keep some matters private.

Pray Honestly

Christians often find themselves in depression when they neglect their quiet time or prayer time. When is the last time you got alone with God and listened for the same still, small voice Elijah heard? God used the thunder, lightning, and earthquakes simply to get Elijah's attention. Could it be that

God is using some crisis in your life to get your attention? I have learned in life to pray honestly to God. In my personal prayers with God, very seldom do I "dress up" my dialogue with the Divine. I simply tell God exactly how I feel. Truly, prayer and meditation is the best mechanism to use when feeling depressed. Prayer not only allows you to dialogue with God but also it allows God to bring clarity to your circumstances. Simply, prayer is talking and listening to God. Prayer is a two-way street and not a one-way road. Again, one of the best things to do when you have depressed thoughts is to simply pray to God and listen for God.

> **PRAY ANYWHERE:** in the wilderness like Hagar, in the streets like Jairus, in your bed like Hezekiah (Just pray!)
> **PRAY ANYHOW:** short like the publican, long like Job, quiet like Hannah, (Just pray!)
> **PRAY FOR ANYTHING:** mercy like David, rain like Elijah, help like Jonah (Just pray!)
> **PRAY ANY TIME:** in the morning like David, at noon like Daniel, at midnight like Silas (Just pray!)

Expect Discouragement but enjoy the journey

In the words of William Ward, "Discouragement is dissatisfaction with the past, distaste for the present, and distrust of the future. It is ingratitude for the blessings of yesterday, indifference to the opportunities of today, and insecurity regarding strength for tomorrow. It is unawareness of the presence of beauty, unconcern for the needs of our fellowman, and unbelief in the promises of old. It is impatience with time, immaturity of thought, and impoliteness to God." Apostle James teaches us that trials, test, and temptations will come to test our faith and patience. However, trouble is a God-magnet. Every time redeemed people or nations find themselves in trouble,

God is there to help them through it. In short, expect discouragement but do not become discouraged.

God's promise to Apostle Paul in Second Corinthians 12:9 says, "My grace is sufficient for thee: for my strength is made perfect in weakness." Warren Weirsbe says, "God did not give Apostle Paul any explanations. Instead, He gave him a promise. We do not live on explanations; we live on promises." In other words, God was going to bless Apostle Paul with whatever he needed to both endure and live the Christian life. God's promise was a sure thing for Apostle Paul and it is for us as well. We must believe things are going to get better. We must trust in the One who can make things better. Keeping yourself out of sight and putting Jesus Christ in full view can be a helpful strategy for you. Indeed, we must get our mind off ourselves and get it on Christ and others. I have learned the more I love Jesus and others, the less depressed I am.

Depression, I have been there. I second that emotion!

SMALL GROUP DISCUSSION QUESTIONS:

1. List five instances in which you were depressed.

2. Write a short sentence prayer that expresses your depressed emotions to God.

3. What strategies did you employ to help you deal with your depression? Do you believe that you utilized healthy strategies? Please explain.

4. Do you, in some ways, identify with Elijah's depressed state? How?

5. Do you believe that embracing Biblical hope will help you recover from depression? Why or why not?

Grief

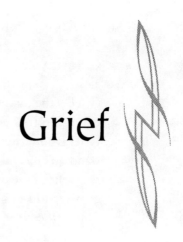

Scriptural Spotlight: Saint John 11:35

"Jesus wept."

GRIEF IS DIFFICULT, *isn't it?* Grief is not a sporting event that ends at the click of the stop watch. Grief is not a mountain climbing exhibition whereby the strong reaches the top before the weak does. Grief comes to anyone who has loss something or someone of value. Grief can slow you down and stop you dead in your tracks. As a matter of fact, everyone grieves.

WHAT IS GRIEF?

The **Grief Recovery Institute** defines grief as "not just sadness, but a *normal* response to the loss of any significant object or person." Any loss can bring about grief: divorce, retirement, loss of wages, loss of a loved one, loss of a contest, loss of health, even the loss of confidence.

I Second that Emotion

Author Edgar Jackson poignantly describes grief:

- Grief is a young widow trying to raise her three children, alone.
- Grief is the man so filled with shocked uncertainty and confusion that he strikes out at the nearest person.
- Grief is a mother walking daily to a nearby cemetery to stand quietly and alone a few minutes before going about the tasks of the day. She knows that part of her is in the cemetery, just as part of her is in her daily work.
- Grief is the silent, knife-like terror and sadness that comes a hundred times a day, when you start to speak to someone who is no longer there.
- Grief is the emptiness that comes when you eat alone after eating with another for many years.
- Grief is teaching yourself to go to bed without saying good night to the one who has died.
- Grief is the helpless wishing that things were different when you know they are not and never will be again.
- Grief is a whole cluster of adjustments, apprehensions, and uncertainties that make it difficult to redirect our energies to move forward.

HOW SHOULD I GRIEVE?

In reality, grief is as unique as your fingerprint. No two people grieve alike. We grieve each loss in a manner unique to that loss.

> No one really knows how long you should grieve

No one really knows how long you should grieve. No one, on Earth, has a magical answer to take your grief away. A grieving person must allow him or herself to face and experience grief in order to begin the journey toward healing.

46

HOW DO I KNOW THAT I AM GRIEVING?

1. Do you feel that you are no longer valuable as a person?
2. Do you speak of the deceased in the present tense?
3. Have you moved from social to anti-social behavior?
4. Do you awaken in the morning feeling fatigued and face the day with dread?
5. Do you find yourself thinking about your own death, wishing life were over or that you are afraid you might commit suicide?
6. Do you breathe irregularly, sigh repeatedly, and feel "heavy in the chest?
7. Do you express a refusal to change the deceased person's room or closet?
8. Do you or others detect that you are becoming irritable?
9. Do you find yourself playing the "Only If" or "If I Would Have" mental game?
10. Do you have great trouble being enthusiastic about anything?

If you answered YES to most of the above questions, chances are you are grappling with grief.

There are a number of Biblical characters that dealt with grief.

A short list includes:

Moses (Exodus 32:32)
Job (Job 3:1, 17:1)
Jonah (Jonah 4:3)
Jeremiah, The Weeping Prophet (Jeremiah 20:18)
The Lord Jesus Christ (Saint John 11:35, Isaiah 53:3)
Joseph (Genesis 50:3)

As you read and study each Biblical character, which one do you more closely resemble? Why?

_____

_____

_____

_____

_____

_____

_____

CAN THERE BE "GOOD GRIEF"?

One of my favorite cartoon characters is Charlie Brown. Charlie Brown had a knack for expressing himself. One of his favorite expressions was "Good Grief." What is good grief? Is good grief possible? I am not sure what Charlie Brown meant, but I can tell you what Jesus means. Jesus has changed the meaning of grieving. There are many people who grieve without any hope for the future. For many, loss is like a period at the end of a sentence. It is a complete and final action. For the believer, loss is a comma. It is a brief pause in action. We must recognize the pause, breathe, and continue on. Early in Jesus' ministry, he explained grieving to us. One part of the Sermon on the Mount found in Saint Matthew 5:4 says, "Blessed are they that mourn, for they shall be comforted." In Jesus' eyes, grief can be a positive experience because it is mentioned among other positive experiences mentioned in Saint Matthew chapters five through seven. Grief is a gift and a growing experience from God. My mother and father bought many gifts that I did not appreciate fully until I was much older. Well, that it is also true in the spiritual world. Grief is a gift! While going through our grieving experience, we must realize that God is not trying to HURT us rather His desire is to HEAL us. Grief allows us to cry and contemplate. While grieving, one good cry may not be enough to soothe your wounded soul. However, the gift of grief helps us to cry, then move on to a greater revelation of the all-sufficiency of God. One well-known speaker suggested that with grief you must **move on** with your life. You must **move beyond** painful emotions of hurt and despair. You have to learn to **move around**, meet new people, and enjoy new experiences. Finally, you must **move up** in your faith to trust God and believe that He will fill the void in your life. Grief is a gift because it helps us to **move to a new level** of dependence in God.

In your opinion, what makes grief a positive experience?

_____

_____

_____

_____

_____

_____

GRIEF INVOLVES READJUSTING

I am an avid evening news watcher. One event that sticks out in my mind was when a storm blew into our city and knocked out the cable. I could hear the voice on the television but I could not see the picture. Therefore, I had to get up and hook on the old antenna. Once I made this readjustment, I could see clearly what I was hearing. In life, storms will come and place you in dark situations. Be aware that there are moments in life when you must make adjustments in order to see and hear from God clearly.

A SUGGESTED METHOD TO DEAL WITH GRIEF

Once again, a grieving person must allow him or herself to face and experience grief in order to begin the journey toward healing. Allow me to share with you my own personal formula in dealing with grief. My personal opinion is that an individual never fully overcomes grief until Heaven. I believe that is why the *Bible* is descriptive when it tells us in Revelation 21:4 "And God shall wipe away all tears from their eyes; and there shall be no more death, neither sorrow, nor crying, neither shall there be any more pain: for the former things are passed away." However, I firmly believe that we can get a grip on our grief so that we can remain productive people on this planet. My suggested method in dealing with grief is to help somebody else who is going through the grieving process. Nothing brings more satisfaction in this life than sacrificial giving. The Acts 20:35 principle of "it is more blessed to give than to receive" was stressed by Jesus in both His life and His words. Without question, giving while grieving can be an antidote for you. The story is told of a woman who was suffering with grief. She went to her pastor for spiritual guidance. Her pastor told her to go to all the homes within one mile of the church to see if she could find one person who was not suffering in some form. As the suffering woman went to visit each home, she discovers that each residence is dealing with some form of suffering. As she listens to each story, she begins to minister and share possible solutions with them. When this woman arrives back to the church, she is smiling. The pastor begins to grin as well. The woman said, "Pastor, I feel so much better by helping others even though my problems have not been worked out." The pastor smiled and responded, "Amen. You are looking at a person who uses this method everyday." The woman gasped and then left with a greater appreciation of the Gospel message and her minister. Without question, serving others while suffering can be a helpful solution for you.

Do you believe helping others while at the same time you need help can be a healthy solution as you deal with your grief? Why or why not?

_____

_____

_____

_____

_____

_____

Here is how to be a giving person while grieving—

BE THERE

During times of grief, most people do not remember the words you say to them. However, they do remember that you were there. Our job is to become conduits of healing whereby we live out the commandments of Christ to care for one another.

The *Bible* shares with us several "one another" commands, such as:

- First John 4:7, "Beloved, let us love one another: for love is of God; and every one that loveth is born of God, and knoweth God."
- Saint John 13:35, "By this shall all men know that ye are my disciples, if ye have love one to another."
- First Peter 4:9, "Use hospitality one to another without grudging."
- Hebrews 3:13, "But exhort one another daily, while it is called Today; lest any of you be hardened through the deceitfulness of sin."

LISTEN

One profitable business in Kansas City, Missouri is a "call me up and I will listen to you" company. This corporation charges a nominal fee to listen to you talk. From what I understand, it has become a very lucrative practice in our city. It seems that people desire to be around others who will intently listen. A grieving person needs to talk in detail about the feelings that he or she is experiencing. When grieving persons talk of their experiences it generally loosens the inner struggles that seem to be keeping them from continuing to enjoy a fulfilling and rewarding life.

USE GOD'S WORD TO COMFORT

We are called to be ministers of hope. At the same time, we can be overwhelmingly unsympathetic while we believe we are being ultra-spritual. One thing we must do is to avoid the temptation to use *killer cliches* and utilize God's word as a helpful tool in the grieving process. Killer cliches are sayings such as:

"Time will heal your wounds."

"You will feel better in the morning."
"There is a silver lining on every dark cloud."

These statements may be well-meant; however, they mean very little to a grieving person in the midst of their deep emotional experiences.

A short list of scriptures to read and share while an individual who is going through the painstaking realities of grief is one effective way to help such as Psalm 116:15, Isaiah 57:1–2, and Revelation 14:13.

HELP THE PERSON FACE HIS OR HER FEELINGS

One of the names of God is Immanuel. Immanuel means "God is with us." In fact, in all of life's successes and sufferings God is a constant companion through each phase. We must help the grieving person understand that it is natural to feel anger, hurt, and pain and that God understands those feelings according to Isaiah 53: 3–5. We must reassure them confidently that God can still calm the seas of our deepest emotional wounds. Furthermore, admitting how we truly feel will help to prevent those unhealthy emotions from festering and nurturing within us.

HELP THE PERSON RE-PRIORITIZE

Grief will cause you to reprioritize your lifestyle. In our fast-paced society, it is relatively easy to lose focus and stray away from the desired path. When tragedy strikes, it causes us to re-evaluate our plans and purpose. One of my favorite stories is about a professor who wanted to explain to his class with crystal clarity the importance of putting "first things first." The professor stood before his philosophy class with several items displayed.

When the class began, wordlessly, he picked up a very large and empty mayonnaise jar and proceeded to fill it with golf balls. He then asked the students if the jar was full. They agreed that it was. The professor then picked up a box of pebbles and poured them into the jar. He shook the jar lightly. The pebbles rolled into the open areas between the golf balls. He then asked the students again if the jar was full. They agreed it was.

The professor next picked up a box of sand and poured it into the jar. Of course, the sand filled up everything else. He asked once more if the jar was full. The students responded with a unanimous "yes."

"Now," said the professor, as the laughter subsided, "I want you to recognize that this jar represents your life. The golf balls are the important things—God, family, your children, your health, and your friends. The pebbles are the other things that matter like your ministry, job, house, and your car. The sand is everything else or the small stuff.

"If you put the sand into the jar first," he continued, "there is no room for the pebbles or the golf balls. The same goes for life. If you spend all your time and energy on the small stuff, you will never have room for the things that are important.

Grief causes you to re-evaluate, re-adjust, and re-prioritize life. The loss of someone or something precious will force us to re-evaluate our goals and aspirations. It will also make us re-adjust to life in our present reality.

Finally, we must reach a point to re-prioritize our value system and begin to place a stronger emphasis on God and Biblical principles and practices.

Grief, I have been there. I second that emotion.

SMALL GROUP DISCUSSION QUESTIONS:

1. List five instances when you grieved.

2. Write a short sentence prayer that expresses your loss to God.

3. What strategies did you employ to help you deal with your grief? Do you believe that you utilized healthy strategies? Please explain.

4. Do you believe that grief is a normal response experienced by the faith and non-faith community? Please explain.

5. Do you believe the author's suggested method in dealing with grief can be a strategy for you? Why or why not?

Guilt

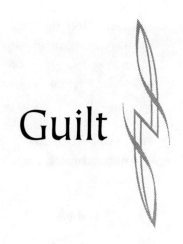

Scriptural Spotlight: Saint Luke 15:21

"And the son said unto him, Father, I have sinned against heaven, and in thy sight, and am no more worthy to be called thy son."

IN EDGAR ALLAN Poe's story, *The Tell-Tale Heart,* the main character committed murder. Unable to escape the haunting guilt of his deed, he begins to hear the heartbeat of the victim he has buried. A cold sweat covers him as he hears the beat-beat-beat of a heart that goes on relentlessly. Ultimately, the heartbeat drives the man insane. Ironically, the heartbeat was not coming from the body beneath the floor but from the heart within his chest. This story helps to teach us about the painstaking realities of guilt. Most researchers define guilt as a heavy-laden heart and an unforgiving conscience.

For example, on the dashboard of my vehicle, the warning sign flashes this message SERVICE THE ENGINE. The only thing wrong with this warning is that the engine has been serviced, but there is a malfunction in my vehicle that will not allow the warning sign to stop flashing each time my car is in motion. Does this sound like you? Do you feel like every time you try to move on with your life, a constant reminder of your former self keeps reoccurring?

Many people in their wedded life, work life, and worship life deal with guilt. Every where you go you will meet, some times unknowingly, Mr. or Ms. Busted, Disgusted, and cannot seem to be Trusted. Quite simply, guilt lies within the heart of princes, paupers, preachers, parents, politicians, and every day people.

- Is there any help for the guilty?
- Is there a process or plan to aid those who are dealing with guilty feelings?

Our discovery must first begin with a proper understanding of the meaning of guilt.

WHAT IS GUILT?

James J. Messina, Ph.D. of Tampa, Florida defines guilt as:

- a feeling of responsibility for negative circumstances that have befallen yourself or others.
- a feeling of regret for your real or imagined misdeeds, both past and present.
- a sense of remorse for thoughts, feelings, or attitudes that were or are negative, uncomplimentary, or non-accepting concerning yourself or others.
- a feeling of bewilderment and lack of balance for not responding to a situation in your typical, stereotype manner.
- a feeling of loss and shame for not having done or said something to someone who is no longer available to you.

- accepting the responsibility for someone else's misfortune or problem because it bothers you to see that person suffer.

In many instances, guilt is a feeling of constant condemnation after an immoral situation. In my years of pastoral experience, I have discovered that people can be obsessed by the memory of some sin or failure committed years ago. It never leaves them. It haunts them. The trauma of the past cripples their ministry, fractures their devotional life, and barricades their relationships with others. They live in constant fear that someone will discover their past. They work overtime trying to prove to God that they are repentant. Friends, do not let that be your "final answer." Unless we experience the truth in First John 3:19– 20 "for if our heart condemn us, God is greater than our heart, and knoweth all things." In other words, the writer of this text helps us to understand that God is greater than our conscience. Until we come to grips with this truth, we will never experience the freedom that grace provides. Instead of being hung up about our past, we ought to rejoice that God has allowed us to outlast our past and create a brand new destiny!

Studies reveal that there are three types of guilt.

Social guilt occurs when a person violates the social expectations of other people in his or her society. This kind of person usually behaves rudely, gossips maliciously, and criticizes unkindly.

Personal guilt occurs when an individual violates his or her own personal standards. For example, guilt may emerge if church is important to you and business has you away on Sundays.

Theological guilt occurs when we violate the true standards of God. Let me add that when we sin, we are guilty of the standards of God whether we feel remorseful or not.

Have you ever experienced any of these types of guilt? Which type? How did you feel?

_____

_____

_____

_____

_____

_____

THE MORAL, PHYSICAL, AND SPIRITUAL IMPLICATIONS OF GUILT

Guilt is a moral issue as well as a spiritual issue and often arises from moral/spiritual failures. Guilt can also bring about physical problems. Guilt can lead to insomnia, loud outbursts, anxiety, and an attitude that displays a harsh criticism toward others.

To deal with guilt it takes more than values, vernacular, and Valium. It takes the veracity of the Word of God. Guilt must be unlocked from deep within so an individual can experience the freedom that comes from having a fruitful fellowship with our Heavenly Father.

THERE IS A BLESSING IN BEING BUSTED

God has unique ways in dealing with waywardness. One strategy the Lord will employ

> There is a blessing in being caught because it generally leads to conversion

when He cannot get your attention through Bible study, sermons, and other people is to gain your undivided attention through pain. Most assuredly, if God cannot get your attention with a whisper, He will throw a brick through your window and shatter your glass. Even though, you have to "pay" for the glass shattered, you will one day thank God for the pain that brought forth your new pane. Oh yes, out of pain God will give you a new pane! One of the first things that I try to convey to people who have guilt feelings in terms of indiscretion and painful incidences is that you ought to rejoice that you were caught.

Does that sound strange to you?

- In Second Samuel chapter 12, God was bringing honor to King David by being caught!
- In Saint Matthew chapter 14, Peter was glad that he was caught in his lies because he found out that he had little faith.
- In Saint John chapter 4, Jesus was bringing honor to the woman by revealing her indiscretions!
- In Acts 6: 11–15, Stephen is glad that he was caught because when he was captured his capturers saw the face of an angel.
- In Acts 16: 19–30, Paul and Silas are glad they were caught so the keeper of the prison could find God.

There is a blessing in being caught because it generally leads to conversion. It is a painful experience to have to endure. However, if you can take it you can really make it.

COUNSELING THE GUILTY

Second Corinthians 7: 10 states, "For godly sorrow worketh repentance to salvation not to be repented of: but the sorrow of the world worketh death." This passage provides the key to leading people to a place of repentance without creating guilt feelings. In this key verse, Apostle Paul contrasts worldly sorrow against godly sorrow. Worldly sorrow brings on self-criticism and self-condoning but godly sorrow leads to constructive change. Moreover, when you are truly sorry for your sins, you will cease doing those things that you used to do that brought about this expressed guilt.

CONSOLING AND CONNECTING WITH THE GUILTY

The attitude of Jesus in dealing with the woman at the well shows us how to console the guilty. In dealing with the woman at the well, Jesus did not **CONDONE** her sin, but he did **CONSOLE** her by stating, "Go, and sin no more."

In fact, in Saint John 8:1–9, there is a key principle that we ought to illuminate. Notice again that Jesus does not **CONDONE** her sin, but he did **CONSOLE** her. One preacher noted that we ought to be glad that Jesus wrote her indiscretion in the sand and not in cement. If Jesus had written the statement in cement it would be still be there. God does not cement our calamity. When we confess our sins, God sends a wind from Heaven that will wipe away whatever we have done. ***Hallelujah!***

CONCLUSIONS ABOUT GUILT

When Jesus talked to the woman caught in adultery, He never relaxed his standards. God's standards are perfect and He never settles for imperfection. The woman was told to sin no more that means that Jesus expected some radical improvements.

What radical improvements do you need to make in your life?

_____

_____

_____

_____

_____

_____

_____

Do you believe that having an accountability partner (a person you can pray and share things with openly and honestly) could be a solution for you? Why or Why not?

_____

_____

_____

_____

_____

_____

In short, we cannot change what we have done. However, we can do something about what we have done. We must take our imperfections and with God's help begin to make marked improvements.

CONQUERING GUILT

As a boy, I remember the church singing a hymn that had these words, "lose all our GUILT and stain." How can you lose all of your guilt? Is it possible for guilt to dissolve? Utilizing the acrostic of GUILT by a well-known author will help us better understand this point.

Get God's grace

What is grace? When a person works an eight-hour day and receives a fair day's pay for his time that is a wage. When a person competes with an opponent and receives a trophy for his performance that is a prize. However, when a person is not capable of earning a wage, cannot win a prize, and deserves no award—yet receives such a gift anyway—that is a good picture of God's unmerited favor. This is the grace of God! We do not deserve God's grace nor can we work to achieve it. Grace is God's undeserved favor. In short, *you cannot pay your sin debt!* Reading an extra chapter in the *Bible* will not repay your sin debt. Praying an extra ten minutes each night will not repay your sin debt.

Grace is extended freely to all that will receive it.

Grace is the atoning work of Jesus Christ on the cross.

Grace is given to all believers of Jesus Christ.

Grace is extended to all believers who desire to repent of their actions. Once again, repentance (godly sorrow) will lead to constructive change. Repentance is more than saying, "I am sorry I was caught." Repentance says, "I am sorry enough to quit the sinful or shameful action or activity." How can you receive God's grace? If you do not have a relationship with Jesus Christ, ask God to forgive you of your sins and come into your heart by praying and believing the scripture found in Romans 10: 9–10. If you are a follower of Jesus, pray the prayer found in Psalm 51: 1–10 then read and meditate on First John chapter 1.

These scriptures will bring restoration into your heart, soul, and spirit as you seek to live for God in a renewed mindset.

How long will you allow guilt feelings to enslave you?

U go to God

I heard a story about a little boy who was visiting his grandparents that helps to illuminate and bring into focus this point. This little boy received a slingshot as a gift from his grandparents.

> How long will you allow guilt feelings to enslave you?

Being grateful of his gift, he practiced in the woods, but he could never hit his target. He went back to Grandma's back yard, where he spotted her pet duck. On an impulse, he took aim. The stone hit, and the duck fell dead.

The boy panicked. Desperately he hid the dead duck in the woodpile, only to look up and see his sister watching. Sally had seen it all, but she said nothing. After lunch that day, Grandma said, "Sally, let's wash the dishes."

However, Sally said, "Johnny told me he wanted to help in the kitchen today. Didn't you, Johnny?" Moreover, she whispered to him, "Remember the duck! Therefore, Johnny did the dishes.

Later Grandpa asked if the children wanted to go fishing. Grandma said, "I'm sorry, but I need Sally to help make supper." Sally smiled and said, "That's all taken care of. Johnny wants to do it." Again, she whispered, "Remember the duck." Johnny stayed while Sally went fishing.

After several days of Johnny doing both his chores and Sally's, finally he could not stand it. He confessed to Grandma that he had killed the duck. "I know, Johnny," she said, giving him a hug. "I was standing at the window and saw the whole thing. Because I love you, I forgave you. I wondered how long you would let Sally make a slave of you.

*Have you done anything that has brought about a sense of regret?
What will you begin to do to change the way you feel?*

_____

_____

_____

_____

_____

_____

_____

*Do you believe sin can enslave you? If so, list certain areas in
your life where you need freedom and healing.*

_____

_____

_____

_____

_____

_____

_____

I must go to God right now through Jesus Christ

Hebrews 4:14–16 states, "Seeing then that we have a great
high priest, that is passed into the heavens, Jesus the Son of
God, let us hold fast our profession. For we have not an high
priest which cannot be touched with the feeling of our infirmities;
but was in all points tempted like as we are, yet without sin. Let

us therefore come boldly unto the throne of grace, that we may obtain mercy, and find grace to help in time of need." This passage teaches us that we have an Advocate presently, positionally, and powerfully. Jesus is there to help you right now **(presently)**. Jesus Christ has face-to-face access to the Father, which enables Him to speak for us in our time of need **(positionally)**. Jesus is our sympathetic friend who has defeated every earthly challenge known to man **(powerfully)**. However to access the privileges of the Advocate, we must decide to go to Him right now. The longer we delay in going to God, the longer we allow this unhealthy emotion to fester within us.

Learn to seek forgiveness

Forgiveness is choosing to pardon, remit, or overlook the mistake, fault, offense, hurt, or injury of the offender without demanding penalty, punishment, or retribution. Forgiveness is "never free," though it can and should be freely given to others. Forgiveness allows the wrongdoer and the wronged to begin reestablishing a relationship. Forgiving and releasing old hurts and hate from your system is like taking a mental and emotional bath. It allows the dirt, scum, and hidden dust to remove itself from your body. The alternative to forgiveness is, in the end, a ceaseless process of hurt, bitterness, anger, resentment, and self-destruction. We often feel that we deserve to suffer for our own transgressions. This is actually a sign of the sin nature that we possess. When we experience personal pain, we often feel that it is a form of justice for our wrongdoing. Nothing can be further from the truth. In fact, that is a faulty assumption.

The best I can explain forgiveness in the natural realm is by comparing forgiveness to opaque fluid. Opaque fluid is the magical liquid that covers over your errors, your typos, and your unfortunate slip-ups. Opaque fluid advertises that it is an obliteration of a goof with no identifiable traces that the mishap happened at all. In other words, the mistake is the recipient of a cover up. Accepting God's forgiveness makes you a recipient of God's Divine Cover Up! Why do you need God's forgiveness? Your crime against God is like owing him 100 billion dollars, and the only way you could pay him back is by doing good deeds that earns you a penny per good deed. It is much easier to accept the forgiveness that God is so graciously willing to offer you! God's forgiveness pays your sin debt and provides you with a blank page to write a new story for His glory.

Trust that you have been forgiven (It is a FACT and not a feeling)

So often, we fail to embrace the Biblical freedom and forgiveness we receive from God because we are inclined to seek a feeling of restoration. Because we are emotional creatures, one of our greatest drawbacks is that we are always seeking a feeling. Your forgiveness from God is based upon the *facts* of the scriptures and not from the feelings that you are receiving in your present emotional state. Simply, when God forgives we are forgiven. The story that I heard about President James Garfield helps to illuminate this point. James Garfield was a lay preacher and principal of his denominational college. He was ambidextrous and could simultaneously write Greek, with one hand and Latin with the other.

In 1880, he was elected president of the United States. After only six months in office, he was shot in the back with a revolver. Surprisingly, he never lost consciousness. At the hospital, the doctor probed the wound with his little finger to seek the bullet. He could not find it, so he tried a silver-tipped probe. The bullet still could not be located. Therefore, they took Garfield back to Washington, D.C. Despite the summer heat, they tried to keep him comfortable. He was growing very weak. Probing the wound repeatedly, teams of doctors tried to locate the bullet. In desperation, they asked Alexander Graham Bell to see if he could locate the metal inside the president's body. He came, he sought, and he too failed. The president hung on through July, through August, but in September, he finally died. James Garfield's cause of death was not from the wound. His death occurred due to the infection caused by the repeated probing.

The repeated probing, which the physicians thought would help the man, eventually killed him. Dwelling too long on our sins or mistakes and exhibiting a refusal to release can hinder our spiritual walk with Jesus. Repeated probing causes an infection that could lead you further away from restoration. Please remember God forgives and because of this truth, we are forgiven and our guilt is removed. However, we must trust and accept God's forgiveness, then forgive ourselves.

Do you believe dwelling too long on past failures can be a hindrance? Please explain.

_____

_____

_____

_____

_____

_____

What mistake in your life are you probing repeatedly?

_____

_____

_____

_____

_____

_____

_____

GUILT—THE AFTERGLOW

When we transgress or break the laws of God, we are guilty. However, when God forgives us—He removes our guilt. Moreover, when **guilt** is taken out of the word **guilt**y we are still

> **Removing** GUILT **from** GUILTY—**will always leave us with Y (why)**

left with Y (why). Thus, when God removes our guilt, guilt feelings still remain. However, God provides means and mechanisms for us to deal with our guilt feelings. A guilt feeling is the "residue" that is left after the redemptive work of Jesus has taken place in your life. For example, there are a few times when I have the arduous task of washing dishes. Not long ago, I washed all the dishes, but I did not clean out the sink. After putting the dishes in the cupboard, I noticed that there was residue in the sink. The residue in the sink gave witness that some cleaning had taken place. It often seems that when everything is gone, some remnants of guilt remain. Ask God to wipe away the residue. Yes, God can wipe clean the basin of your blunders, the sink of your sin, and the residue of your wrongdoing.

Guilt, I have been there. I second that emotion.

SMALL GROUP DISCUSSION QUESTIONS:

1. List five instances in which you have expressed guilt.

2. Write a short sentence prayer that expresses your guilt feelings to God.

3. What strategies did you employ to help you deal with your guilt? Do you believe that you utilized healthy strategies? Please explain.

4. Do you believe that there is a unique blessing in having a hidden sin exposed? Why or why not?

5. Do you believe that the author's five steps will help you to overcome guilt and guilt feelings? Why or why not?

Loneliness

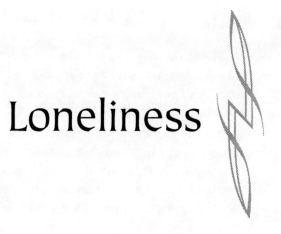

Scriptural Spotlight: Second Timothy 4:10

"For Demas hath forsaken me, having loved this present world, and is departed unto Thessalonica; Crescens to Galatia, Titus unto Dalmatia."

LONELINESS IS LIKE **being in solitary confinement without metal bars.** Recently I attended with my wife and children a Black Church Leadership Conference in Glorieta, New Mexico where a Southern Baptist pastor was making a powerful point about loneliness. He used the example of a group of keys. Each key had its own function and responsibility. The keys were a part of the key ring. When the lock had to be changed on an entrance, one particular key lost its significance, function, and responsibility. However, the key remained a part of the key ring. This key remained with the other keys; however, a lack of significance, function, and responsibility led to loneliness. Every other key felt significant because it could unlock the doors to the building; however, this key had lost its function.

WHAT IS LONELINESS?

Loneliness, as we use the term today, means unwanted, self-conscious, or emotional isolation. Loneliness is a condition in which the lonely one is consciously aware that something important is painfully lacking in his or her life. I call loneliness the UN disease. The prefix UN has a way of handcuffing positive words.

> Loneliness is a signal that something is missing in your life

Generally, any time UN precedes a word—it has a way of turning a positive experience into a pathetic experience.

Loneliness is a feeling of being unneeded, unloved, unwanted, and even unnecessary. It is a desperate sense of "Nobody needs me." "Nobody wants me." "Nobody loves me." **Loneliness says, "I am just not important to this world."**

Have you ever felt unneeded and unloved? What transpired in your life to bring about this feeling?

_____

_____

_____

_____

_____

_____

It is strange to me that in an age when there are more people on earth and more ways to communicate with each other than ever before, people are lonelier. Cities and towns are simply places where thousands of people can be lonely together. High-rise

74

apartments, multi-housing units, manufactured home communities, and area subdivisions are nothing more than monuments of loneliness. A recent Gallop poll said four out of ten Americans admit to frequent feelings of intense loneliness.

Mary Ellen Copeland, M.S. describes loneliness as:

- a feeling of having no common bond with the people around you
- a feeling of disconnection from others
- a feeling of sadness because there is no one else available to be with you
- an uncomfortable feeling of being by yourself
- a feeling that there is no one in your life who really cares about you
- being without friends or a companion
- feeling abandoned
- being unable to connect with anyone on either a physical or emotional level
- feeling left out
- feeling uncomfortable being with yourself

Are any of the above statements indicative of your current emotional state? Which one(s)?

_____

_____

_____

_____

_____

_____

_____

Few emotions are more painful than the emotion of loneliness. The book, *The Purpose Driven Life*, states, "We were formed by God to fellowship with Him and our brothers and sisters." Indeed, people were created with a twofold need—fellowship with God and companionship with other human beings. From reading the book, *The Purpose Driven Life,* we discover that there is a void in our life that can only be filled by having a fruitful and daily fellowship with God on a consistent basis. At the same time, we must challenge ourselves to engage in encouraging companionship with other people. However, loneliness is a grave feeling of disconnection.

- Think of the single person enduring the pain of a broken romance.
- Think of the divorced person who does not know what to do with his or her time over the holidays.
- Think of the inmate behind the bars of solitary confinement.
- Think of the military person overseas.
- Think of the widow whose table is still set for two.
- Think of the parents whose arms ache for a missing child.
- Think of the person who may be around acquaintances everyday but still has no vital connection.

We have all been there—a part of the crowd but not of the community. There is never a time in life when we can completely escape from loneliness. Loneliness can sneak upon all of us.

In what areas of your life do you feel a sense of disconnection?

_____

_____

_____

LONELINESS IS NOT HOMESICKNESS

Loneliness should not be confused with homesickness. God has afforded me to pastor different types of people who express loneliness but in reality, it is homesickness.

- A college student away from home may experience a deep longing to be reunited with his family.
- A soldier stationed overseas has a deep desire to be among friends and family.
- A traveling salesman often feels the magnetic pull to get back to his hometown.

None of these examples defines loneliness. They authentically affirm the definition of homesickness, but not loneliness.

LONELINESS IS NOT A SIN

Loneliness is not a sin. Loneliness is a signal that something is missing in your life.

Ultimately, loneliness stems from humankind's alienation from God. Unless this area is addressed, you may only discover superficial and temporary relief. Numbers 11:14–17 states, "I am not able to bear all this people alone, because it is too heavy for me. And if thou deal thus with me, kill me, I pray thee, out of hand, if I have found favour in thy sight; and let me not see my wretchedness. And the LORD said unto Moses, Gather unto me seventy men of the elders of Israel, whom thou knowest to be the elders of the people, and officers over them; and bring them unto the tabernacle of the congregation, that they may stand there with thee. And I will come down and talk with thee there: and I will take of the spirit which is upon thee, and will put it upon them; and they shall bear the burden of the people with thee, that thou bear it not thyself alone." When Moses makes this declaration unto God, he was feeling the intense feeling of being alone. Not only did Moses need reassurance that people would support him; moreover, he wanted to know that God would be with him throughout the process.

DEFEATING LONELINESS THROUGH SOLITUDE

Defeating loneliness occurs when you create a healthy balance between being with others and being alone. Solitude is a predetermined plan to spend quality time with the Savior of the world. One key ingredient to add to your solitude moment is silence. Without silence, there is no solitude. Richard Foster's book *Celebration of Discipline* says, "these two things, silence and solitude, are as connected and inseparable as peanut butter and jelly." I sincerely advocate for any believer to have some "alone" time with God every day. When is the last time you spent some time alone with God?

It was while alone with God that:

Adam and Eve saw the guilt of their disobedience

Abraham proved his love for God on Mt. Moriah

Jacob wrestled with an angel and was blessed

Enoch walked with God and was raptured

> Sometimes we do not recognize that God is all we need until God is all we have.

Moses received the Ten Commandments on Mt. Sinai
Hannah was promised a son would be born unto her

It was while alone with God that:

Elijah prayed down fire and the rain
Elisha smote the Jordan and passed through on dry ground
Hezekiah received fifteen more years of life
Daniel slept peacefully in the lion's den
Moses saw the bush that burned with fire
Aaron sprinkled the blood upon the Mercy Seat
Gideon was called to be the leader of his people
Ezekiel witnessed the glory of God

It was while alone with God, that:

Elijah heard the still small voice
Mary conceived within her the Son of God
Jesus prayed in the Garden of Gethsemane
Mary Magdalene saw the resurrected Lord in the Garden
John received the Revelation of end time events
Everyone should devote some time in his or her daily schedule to be alone with God!

How much time can you devote to spending quiet time with God on a daily basis? How has it helped you?

_____

_____

_____

_____

_____

_____

MOVING FROM HOME ALONE TO MAKING IT BACK HOME!

A Japanese sculptor came to America with a unique twist on his art. At his exhibit, each piece had a small sign that read, "Please touch." He literally wanted people to feel his art. Loneliness causes you to wear an invisible sign around your neck that says, "Do not touch." Because loneliness is often described as a need to get back home, an illustration of a baseball diamond can aid us in our discovery.

THE BASES TO COVER IN OVERCOMING OUR LONELINESS:

In this ballpark, no doubles, triples, or homeruns are allowed. You must run the bases, one at a time, to make it home.

To get on first base, you must realize that Jesus loves you. He loves you more than the most significant person in your life loves you. Jesus knows you better than anyone else, yet He still loves you more than anyone else.

> JESUS
> LOVES
> YOU

Jeremiah 23:23 states, "Am I a God at hand, saith the LORD, and not a God afar off? Can any hide himself in secret places that I shall not see him? saith the LORD. Do not I fill heaven and earth? saith the LORD." Quite simply, God knows everything about us yet He still loves us.

Are you willing to accept this kind of love? How will go about accepting it?

_____

_____

_____

_____

_____

You move from first base to second base when you understand that Jesus accepts you. Before you ever accepted Jesus in your life, Jesus had already accepted you according to the scripture found in Romans 5:8. Jesus understands your loneliness because He experienced bitter loneliness as identified in

JESUS AC-CEPTS YOU

Saint Luke 9:58. Because of these profound truths, He understands you, and He is willing to accept you into His family. No longer do you have to feel like you do not fit or belong, you can become a vital part of the greatest family in the world—God's family.

Are you willing to accept His acceptance of you? How will go about accepting it?

_____

_____

_____

_____

_____

_____

You can move from second base to third base when you fully embrace the fact that Jesus needs you! You can be a member of a winning team that gives heavenly rewards and is full of eternal benefits. You can join God in performing a ministry and sharing the good news of Jesus Christ with others. Please recall that loneliness is a deep desire to feel needed, wanted, and connected.

JESUS NEEDS YOU

Are you willing to accept His invitation to join Him in His work? How will go about accepting it?

_____

_____

_____

_____

_____

_____

How can we make it to home plate, pastor? You may be thinking, "I need somebody real. I need somebody who IS here, right now!" In the words of the late Dr. E.K. Bailey of Concord Baptist Church of Dallas, Texas, "Too many Christians are stuck on third base!" Until you understand that Jesus Christ IS real and that Jesus IS here right now, you will never conquer your loneliness nor make it home to happiness, health, and harmony. You must affirm that Jesus Christ IS more real than this book in your hand.

A famous pop star, wrote a song with these words: "You are not alone for I am here with you. This singer may not have been trying to convey this eternal truth but it is indicative of the omnipresence of God. God is an ever-present help! In fact, God is my Paraclete! Para means that God is "next to me, right along beside me." Loneliness cannot loom when you fully discover that the Lord is your **PARA**!

He is my:

PARABLE - He gives me a clear understanding.
PARACHUTE - He catches me before I hit rock bottom.
PARADOX - When it seems like things are going LEFT, God makes them go RIGHT.
PARALEGAL - He is my lawyer in the courtroom
PARAMEDIC - He is my doctor in the sickroom
PARALLEL - He leads me in the path of righteousness

In fact, God through Jesus Christ has prepared a place for all people who love Him, which we affectionately call a **PARADISE**.

When loneliness sets in on me from time to time, I have learned to hum the words of that old traditional gospel song, *No Never Alone*. "No never alone, no never alone, He promised never to leave me—no never to leave me alone. Amen.

Loneliness, I have been there. I second that emotion!

SMALL GROUP DISCUSSION QUESTIONS:

1. List five instances that caused you to feel lonely.

2. Write a short sentence prayer that expresses your lonely feelings to God.

3. What strategies did you employ to help you deal with your loneliness? Do you believe that you utilized healthy strategies? Please explain.

4. Have you ever felt like the key on the key ring with no purpose? Please explain.

5. Do you believe that the author's solution of learning how to spend alone time with God will help you in your loneliness? Why or why not?

Stress

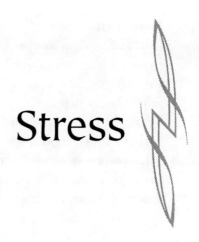

Scripture Spotlight: Second Corinthians 4: 8

"We are troubled on every side, yet not distressed; we are perplexed, but not in despair"

NOT LONG AGO in a respected newspaper, there was a picture of a beautiful brand new home. This large house had a manicured lawn complete with shrubbery and an automatic sprinkler system. The front-page picture showed vivid images of the beauty on the outside, but the caption told the true story on the inside. For within these walls were dead people. This beautiful house contained the remains of victims of a mass suicide. The outside of the house was beautiful, but the inside was blemished. Related to this story, we live amongst many people who are manicured and sculptured (on the outside); however, stress is destroying them on the inside.

According to the **Saint Luke's Hospital—Heart Institute**, "stress is the non-specific response of the body to any demand placed on it. Stress can create feelings of conflict and/or anxiety within an individual. It can stem from demands one places on oneself or from outside stimuli or situations. Some stress is easily identified, such as increased financial responsibilities; while other stress, such as feeling that one must earn peer acceptance, may go undetected. If stress is not identified and resolved, it can progressively deteriorate one's ability to function." Stress can occur when you are worried about being laid off your job or not having enough money to pay your bills. Stress can also occur when you are worried about your relatives when the doctor says that they may need an operation. In fact, to most of us, stress is synonymous with worry. If it is something that makes you worry, then it could lead to stress.

List a few things in your life that cause you to worry?

_____

_____

_____

_____

_____

_____

Your body, however, has a much broader definition of stress. To your body, stress is synonymous with change. Anything that causes a change, good or bad, in your life causes stress. When you find your dream home and get ready to move, that is stress. If you break your leg, that is stress. Good or bad, if it is a CHANGE in your life, your body may feel stressed.

What lifestyle or job-related changes have occurred in your life within the past year?

_____

_____

_____

_____

_____

_____

_____

The following examples from reputable companies detail for us the harmful effects of stress.

One-fourth of employees view their jobs as the number one stressor in their lives.

—Northwestern National Life

Three-fourths of employees believe the worker has more on-the-job stress than a generation ago.

—Princeton Survey Research Associates

Problems at work are more strongly associated with health complaints than are any other life stressor-more so than even financial problems or family problems.

—St. Paul Fire and Marine Insurance Company

Stress can occur in your place of work, place of worship, and even within your place of residence. The **National Institute for Occupational Safety and Health** (NIOSH) reports that pharmacists prescribe five billion doses of tranquilizers and three billion doses of amphetamines so that people can take

> Why do we seek over the counter answers instead of turning it over to Jesus for our answer?

"the edge off" the damaging effects of stress each year. It seems that everyone is taking "pick me up" or "pull me down" type medication to help them deal with stress.

The Encyclopedia of Occupational Safety and Health reveals the following about stress:

It can lead to cardiovascular disease.
Many studies suggest that psychologically demanding jobs that allow employees little control over the work process increase the risk of cardiovascular disease.

It increases the development of musculoskeletal disorders.
It is widely believed that stress increases the risk for development of back and upper—extremity musculoskeletal disorders.

It can bring about psychological disorders.
Several studies suggest that differences in rates of mental health problems (such as depression and burnout) are due partly to differences in job stress levels.

It can lead to workplace injury.
Although more study is needed, there is a growing concern that stressful working conditions interfere with safe work practices and set the stage for injuries at work.

UNHEALTHY STRESS

Stress can make us increasingly unpleasant. Stress can lead us into developing a pessimistic personality while dealing with our peers, parents, and pastors. It has often been mentioned, "stressing about stuff you have no control over is about as fruitful as trying to put the toothpaste back in the tube." For example, if we do not have a job, we stress about getting a job. If we do have a job, we stress about losing our job. If we do not have a car, we stress about getting a car. If we do have a car, we stress about making the car payments. If we do not have money, we stress about getting some money. If we do have some money, we stress about losing our money. It is so important to realize that stress becomes distress when we feel we cannot handle the pressure or the responsibility. *Consider these passages as it relates to unhealthy stress:*

- Genesis 32:7, Then Jacob was *greatly afraid* and distressed: and he divided the people that was with him, and the flocks, and herds, and the camels, into two bands.
- Judges 10:9, Moreover the children of Ammon passed over Jordan to *fight* also against Judah, and against Benjamin, and against the house of Ephraim; so that Israel was sore distressed.
- First Samuel 30:6, And David was greatly distressed; for *the people spake of stoning him*, because the soul of all the people was grieved, every man for his sons and for his daughters: but David encouraged himself in the LORD his God.

In each instance, something affected them that caused them to experience the harmful effects of stress. Any time you add more onto your normal STRESS BEARING LEVEL it will lead to DISTRESS. The only way STRESS (S-T-R-E-S-S) becomes **DI**STRESS, (D-I-S-T-R-E-S-S) is by adding a little more on to it.

Have you added more assignments or responsibilities to your weekly schedule? When you added these things, do you believe you moved from healthy stress to distress? Please explain?

_____

_____

_____

_____

_____

_____

_____

Easton's Bible Dictionary defines stress as being "drawn tight." When we are stressing, we are really BOUND. In reality, some of us are like Egyptian mummies. Stress always makes you raise the question of "What's binding me?" Are your current problems causing you to feel wrapped tight like an Egyptian mummy?

A mummy is nothing more than a visible expression of the preservation of the dead. A mummy is an upright corpse that is bound. It has an image of life, but what is on the inside is death. A good example of stress is revealed in H. B. London and Neil Wiseman's book *Your Pastor Is An Endangered Species*. It states "Pastors dwell in a world of unfinished tyranny, where they can not shut the door, walk out of the office, or know that something is completely finished. There is always another Bible study, sermon, phone call, committee meeting, hospital call, home visit, or gathering clamoring for attention." Lloyd Rediger in his book, *Clergy Killers*, says that Pastors are ". . . still expected to produce reassuring sermons, exciting programs and manage the church budget without causing discomfort to anyone but himself." According to a study done by Focus on the Family, 50% of ordained ministers across denominational lines are out of the pulpit within 5 years. Fifteen hundred pastors leave the ministry every month in this country." If this is true of God called ministers, what about every day people. Stress is a real problem that needs a real answer.

If you are searching for a stress-free existence, forget it! Everyone talks about returning to a "simpler" way of life, but no one seems to know exactly what that means or how to attain it. Thus, it is impossible to avoid stress in this life. Consider the

> STRESS IS UNAVOID-ABLE

relationship between a rubber band and stress. A rubber band under no tension is loose and worthless. Even so, a person who experiences no stress is usually ineffective. A rubber band is designed to function under tension.

STRESS IN RELATIONSHIPS

Developing stress-reducing strategies in the area of relationships can help us live healthier lives. Whether the relationship is martial, social, or spiritual, stress can develop if we do not apply patience.

Biblical characters dealt with moments of stress:

Adam and Eve had the serpent . . .   Moses had Pharaoh . . .

David had Goliath . . .   Samson had the Philistines . . .

Gideon had the Midianites . . .   Elijah had Jezebel . . .

Daniel had Nebuchadnezzar . . .   Esther had Haman . . .

John the Baptist had Herod . . .   Paul had Nero . . .

Everybody has somebody . . .

Apostle Paul shares with us in Second Corinthians 4:8, "Trouble is on every side."

So, What's troubling you?

- Sometimes, a husband won't LOVE YOU RIGHT.
- Sometimes a wife won't DO RIGHT .
- Sometimes, it's a child that won't ACT RIGHT.
- Sometimes, it's a job that won't TREAT YOU RIGHT.

Too many people feel BOXED IN BY THEIR BURDENS trying to figure out how to escape out of the CUBE of their present CIRCUMSTANCES.

How can we manage stress? Well, stress is not only found in psychology books but also in engineering books. When an architect designs a building, he is careful to calculate the **stress-bearing capabilities** of the structure. In other words, any good engineer knows just how much the building that he built can bear. Our Divine Designer created us with a capacity to handle stress according to Psalm 103:14.

The Holistic Stress Control Institute admonishes us to try at least three practical stress coping skills to reduce our stress level.

1. **Learn to relax your body.** Just a few minutes of peace and quiet each day will give you the ability to assess most challenging situations and to respond in an appropriate manner.
2. **Learn to relax your mind.** Negative or fearful thoughts create more anxiety and stress. Thinking positive about a situation helps reduce stress.
3. **Learn to laugh more.** Laughter really is good medicine. (Proverbs 17:22)

In the midst of all despair, find a reason to be thankful. A woman once approached a man who had a sour look on his face. She encouraged the grumpy man to be thankful. He replied, "Thankful for what? I don't even have enough money to pay my bills!" The woman thought for a moment then said, "Well then, be thankful you are not one of your creditors." We experience so many blessings in life that it is so easy to take them for granted, look at the cloudy side of life and see only darkness and despair. Continuing to think about all that God has done for us, will enable us to begin to thank Him for all He has helped us to overcome.

A SCRIPTURAL SOLUTION FOR STRESSFUL SITUATIONS

Isaiah 40:31 tells us that "They that wait upon the Lord shall **renew** their strength." The word "renew" in Hebrew means, "to exchange."

The first thing that we must realize is that God wants us to exchange our STRESS for His STRENGTH. This is something that we must do! One of the best ways, I deal with stress is to catch a plane and spend four days and three nights on a Caribbean island. I remember my wife and I went to Cozumel. In Cozumel, a Mexican controlled territory, they have exchange centers. An exchange center is a place where a person can exchange their currency for the currency of that particular province. In Cozumel, I could exchange my dollars for pesos. I utilized this strategy because I discovered that the exchange rate was better. In addition, I discovered that at The Exchange Center I could get more Mexican pesos for my American dollars. In Heaven, God has set up an Eternal Exchange Center whereby you can exchange YOUR STRESS and receive more of HIS SUPERNATURAL STRENGTH. Waiting upon the Lord, without stressing, requires true faith. Waiting upon the Lord requires that we believe in the impossible, look for the unseen answers, and hold on to our Biblical hope in times of hopelessness. Waiting on God is being assured, without knowing why or how, that God will take care of us. For example, baby eaglets, in their nest, can do nothing but wait until the mother eagle returns to her nest to bring the necessary provision. We must stay in the "nest" of God's house, trust in the fact that He will bring us what we need, and then accept and digest what comes because we know its for our own good.

God provides strength over stress in three ways:

1. STRENGTH TO SOAR
   Perhaps you have faced times of intense difficulty when your problems rose up before you like a mighty storm. On these occasions, God will give you the strength to soar above the storm

   > DO NOT STRESS IN THE STORM!

   of adversity. When the storm comes, the eagle allows its wings to spread so that the wind will lift it above the storm. The eagle does not escape the storm; it simply uses the storm to lift it higher! We must allow our storms to raise us to new levels of dependence in God.

   Storms or difficult situations will do three things for us:

   A. Storms *educate us* on the constant friendship and companionship of God.
   B. Storms *enlarge us* to trust Him more each day.
   C. Storms *expose us* so that we can see the level of our faith and Christian maturity.

2. STRENGTH TO MAINTAIN YOUR STAMINA
   The Christian life is not a 100-meter dash; it is a lifetime
   marathon that demands the patience and pacing of God.
   All of us need more patience. It seems that patience is
   no longer a virtue in our society. We are the society that
   invented fast food, microwaves, the Concorde jet, the
   drive-through, pizza delivery in thirty minutes or less,
   and express check-out lanes. Isaiah 40:29–31 really
   makes us think about life. In reality, what can you do
   when you are about to faint physically. You cannot DO
   anything! In your weakness, you fall upon the shoulders
   of some strong loved one, lean hard, and rest until your
   strength returns. The same is true in our relationship
   with Jesus Christ. When life seems to burden us, we can
   depend upon the promises of the scriptures to sustain
   us.

3. STRENGTH TO KEEP ON STRUTTING
   Walking with the Lord does five things for me:

   > *It makes me more forbearing and forgiving of
   > others.*
   > *It energizes me to serve God.*
   > *It increases my respectful appreciation for those
   > who walk with God.*
   > *It increases my love for my Lord.*
   > *It makes me more aware of my shortcomings.*

   There are only a few times in our lives when we are
   required to soar like an eagle; however, we need strength
   to walk each day. Furthermore, we need confidence in
   every day situations to help us reduce our stress levels.
   Saint Matthew 11: 28–30 states, "Come unto me, all ye
   that labour and are heavy laden, and I will give you rest.
   Take my yoke upon you, and learn of me; for I am meek

and lowly in heart: and ye shall find rest unto your souls. For my yoke is easy, and my burden is light." This word "labour" in the Greek is kopiao . According to *Smith's Bible Dictionary*, this word means "to feel fatigue, by implication to work hard: to bestow labor, toil, to become wearied." Thus, THE YOKE OF REST is afforded to those that "come unto Christ" as they seek rest from their heavy labor and load of sin. J.H. Jowett's book, *The School of Calvary*, summarizes this thought when he mentions, "The fatal mistake for the believer is to seek to bear life's load in a single collar. God never intended man to carry his burden alone. A yoke is a neck harness for two, and the Lord Himself promises to be One of the two. He wants to share the labor of any galling task. The secret of peace and victory in the Christian life is found in putting off the taxing collar of self and accepting the Master's relaxing yoke."

God's yoke is a yoke of:

1. Connection—Yokes are made for two, not one. We were not meant to go through life living apart from God. His yoke fits well and is lighter than the one we have been pulling by ourselves.
2. Direction—The idea of a yoke pictures the forward motion of two connected together. You cannot be yoked to Jesus and go your own way. We must follow Him and His direction for our life.
3. Cooperation—To be yoked together means that we cooperate with Him in His work.
    Which yoke do you believe that you have been under man's or God's? How do you know?

Stress, I have been there. I second that emotion.

I Second that Emotion

SMALL GROUP DISCUSSION QUESTIONS:

1. List five situations or events that caused you to become stressed.

2. Write a short sentence prayer that expresses your stressful feelings to God.

3. What strategies did you employ to help you deal with your stress? Do you believe that you utilized healthy strategies? Please explain.

4. In recent months, how have you handled your storms (antagonizing and uncomfortable moments)? Please explain.

5. Do you believe that the author's scriptural solution for stressful situations can help you? Why or why not?

Wanting to Give Up

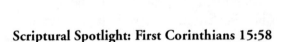

Scriptural Spotlight: First Corinthians 15:58

"Therefore, my beloved brethren, be ye steadfast, unmovable, always abounding in the work of the Lord, forasmuch as ye know that your labor is not in vain in the Lord."

EVERYBODY HAS THOUGHT **about quitting.** Noted author, Gary Enrig, shares the following story about quitting. "The record for the shortest major league baseball career probably belongs to a member of the old Brooklyn Dodgers, a pitcher named Harry Hartman. Harry was a gifted young ballplayer whose day of glory arrived in 1918 when he was called up from the minors to pitch against the Pittsburgh Pirates. This was the moment he had dreamed about, the beginning of a great career, but his dreams began to fade when his first pitch was hit for a single. The next batter tripled. Becoming more frazzled, he walked the next batter on four straight pitches. When he did throw a strike to the next hitter, it went for a single. At that point, Hartman had enough. He headed for the showers, dressed, and walked out of the stadium to a naval recruiting office, where he enlisted. The next day, he was in a military uniform, never to be heard from in professional baseball again." Perhaps, Hartman struggled with the "What's The Use?" syndrome.

Once again, everybody has thought about quitting. Even though many people do not like to admit it, they are suffering from various levels of emotional, spiritual, or mental burnout. When people lose their enthusiasm, excitement, and energy

> Have you ever entertained the thought of "What's The Use?"

in their work, they tend to become bored. Oft times, they begin to reason that it may be time to quit or give up. Yes, even the pastor of your church has probably entertained the thought of "What's The Use?" I am quite sure, from time to time, most people who are in some form of leadership wake up intent on resigning on a Monday morning. In fact, one of the most pervasive spirits in modern day society is a "quitting spirit."

- A "quitting spirit" wants to throw in the towel before the fight is over.
- A "quitting spirit" wants to surrender before the battle is won.
- A "quitting spirit" does not want to keep on keeping on.
- A "quitting spirit" is in the race of faith but lacks the fortitude to see what the end result is going to be.
- A "quitting spirit" desires to take off the garment of praise and armor of God.

Regardless of the well-meant proverb, that states "a winner never quits, and a quitter never wins," everybody has thought about quitting.

- Divorce filings are at an all time high because of this quitting spirit.

- Prisons cannot be built fast enough because of this quitting spirit.
- Adoption centers are at capacity levels with abandoned children because of this quitting spirit.
- Alternative educational schools and systems exist because of this quitting spirit.

From a Biblical perspective, tribes and individuals have entertained thoughts of quitting.

- According to Judges 7, the Midianites made Gideon want to quit.
- According to Judges 15, the Philistines made Samson want to quit.
- According to First Kings 19, Jezebel made Elijah want to quit.
- According to Saint Mark 14:36, even the sins of the world made Jesus want to quit.

Every place you go, you will run into three types of people:

1. Those who are QUESTIONING others about their desire to quit—
2. Those who are in the midst of a QUEST, but at the same time they are thinking about quitting—
3. Those who dealt with the QUESTION of quitting in their minds; however, they did or will not allow it to be their final answer—

The question that must be answered is "Which type are you?" Why do you feel that you fit that type?

_____

_____

_____

_____

_____

_____

_____

Quitting is an easy response to deaden the pain of deferred hope. The cartoon character Charlie Brown builds a beautiful sandcastle. This sandcastle has been worked on by him for many hours. Finally, he stands back and looks at it. Just as he is admiring it, a storm comes up and blows over his entire sandcastle. Now, he is standing where his beautiful masterpiece was, on level sand, saying to himself, "I know there is a lesson in this, but I am not sure what it is." Langston Hughes' poem, *A Dream Deferred*, helps to convey what Charlie Brown experienced.

> What happens to a dream deferred?
> Does it dry up
> like a raisin in the sun?
> Or fester like a sore—
> and then run?
> Does it stink like rotten meat?
> Or crust and sugar over—
> like a syrupy sweet?
> Maybe it just sags
> like a heavy load.
> Or does it explode?

When hopes are dashed and dreams are deferred, the agonizing thoughts of when will it ever happen begins to creep into our minds.

- On our jobs, we wonder when that promotion will ever happen.
- At home, we wonder if the honey that was in the honeymoon will ever happen again.
- At church, we wonder when the spiritual, financial, and numerical growth will ever happen.

Have you gone through any of these antagonizing moments? How did it make you feel?

_____

_____

_____

_____

_____

_____

Moody Bible Institute's *Today in the Word Daily Devotional*, September 5, 1995, uses an illustration that addresses a strategy to utilize when we deal with those dogmatic moments of when "will it ever happen." "While touring Italy, a man visited a cathedral that had been completed on the outside only. Once inside, the traveler found an artist kneeling before an enormous wall upon which he had just begun to create a mosaic. On some tables nearby were thousands of pieces of colored ceramic. Curious, the visitor asked the artist how he would ever finish such a large project. The artist answered that he knew how much he could accomplish in one day. Each morning, he marked off an area to be completed that day. He did not worry about what remained outside that space. That was the best he could do; and if he faithfully did his best, one day the mosaic would be finished." The artist decided to deal with his enormous task by breaking it down into bite-sized chunks. When we get to the point of celebrating small victories, our desire to quit may lessen.

FACTORS THAT LEAD TO EXPRESSING A DESIRE TO GIVE UP

Negative criticism is one of the main ingredients that make people want to quit. There is a difference between criticism and a critique. Most times, people believe that they are offering a critique when actually it is a criticism.

- A criticism is a negative response to a positive outcome.
- A critique is a positive response to a negative outcome.

Since very few people understand the difference, it is fair to suggest that criticism is inevitable. However, how we respond to it makes a huge difference. A seasoned pastor wisely observed: "If your critics control you, you are defeated." Do your critics agitate you to anger, paralyze you with paranoia, intimidate you into inactivity, or simply make you want to quit? How can you deal wisely with critics and their criticism? Whenever you are dealing with criticism, you must ask yourself two questions:

1. What should I learn from the criticism?
2. What action should I take, if any, in response to the criticism?

When I thought about quitting because of a criticism I received from a German Biology professor, I found consolation in a wrinkled up torn out poem that my father gave me as a freshman at Texas A&M University.

When Things Go Wrong

When things go wrong as they sometimes will,
When the road you're trudging seems all uphill,
When the funds are low and the debts are high,
Moreover, you want to smile, but you have to sigh,
When care is pressing you down a bit, Rest if you must,
but do not quit.
So do not give up, though the pace seems slow—For you
may succeed with another blow.
Success is failure, turned inside out, The silver tint of the
clouds of doubt.
And you never can tell how close you are; It may be near
when it seems afar;
So stick to the fight when you're hardest hit,
It's when things seem worst that you must not quit.

Anonymous

It was after reading this poem that I became determined, like Edison who did not quit on the development of the electric light bulb, like Bell who did not quit while developing the telephone, and like Fulton

> Life Challenges us to Change us

who did not quit while developing the steamboat, to develop the fortitude to achieve my goals and dreams with the help of the Lord. Thanks Dad!

Much later in life, I began to embrace the words of the scripture found in First Corinthians 15:58. Apostle Paul shares with us that life CHALLENGES us in order to CHANGE us. In fact, I love thisb scripture so much that I hope the eulogist will preach this text at my Home-going (Funeral) Celebration.

Exodus 15:22 describes how and why Moses wanted to quit. Most times, it is in our most challenging times that we must not quit on God or give up on our goals. As Moses led the children of Israel out of Egypt, he came up against the obstacle of the Red Sea. God supernaturally parted the waters and they passed through to the other side. Furthermore, God used the Red Sea to destroy the enemies who were pursuing the Israelites. However, after a great spiritual victory, Moses still wanted to quit. It happened at a place called Marah. As the Israelites began to travel, they became extremely thirsty. When they came to Marah, they could not drink of its water because it was bitter. Thus, people began to hurl criticism and accusations at Moses. Once again, negative criticism and unjust accusations will make you consider quitting. This passage of scripture teaches us that God did not test them at the Red Sea. Rather, God tested them at Marah. God does not usually test us during times of great spiritual victory, but during episodes of spiritual stress. God is interested to see how we react when we face difficult and discouraging circumstances and people. Again, Apostle Paul's admonition holds true. Life challenges us in order to change us, not destroy us. Life challenges us to lift our hands to God, not throw up our hands and quit.

Three keys can help to unlock us from the room of discouragement or wanting to quit.

Key number one is in our understanding that warfare always surrounds the birth of a miracle. The late and great philosopher Frederick Douglass once said, "Where there is no struggle, there is no progress." This is probably one of the most profound statements ever uttered. Every positive step will be met with negative statements; however, you must have the fortitude to stay with the process and trust in the promise that God made to you. You must remember that God wants you to triumph over every trial, trouble, and tribulation that invades your life. The word triumph has an important meaning within it. The first three letters point out to us that we

> Use
> The Keys
> Saint
> Matthew
> 16:19

must first TRY. The last four letters reveal to us that we must have some UMPH. Triumph will come to the individual who is willing to TRY and who has the UMPH or tenacity in difficult times to stay with it.

Key number two is in the realization that all men fall, but great men get up. Saying "I quit" is an easy choice with an expensive price tag. Quitting allows the dream to perish. One of the most profound places in the entire world is the cemetery. For within the cemetery are many great ideas which have been buried and will never be revealed. You may have fallen from greatness, but you can get up. Great people can overcome every problem and obstacle. The key is learning to continue in the face of opposition and developing the skills to thrive while the crowd cries and complains!

Key number three is in comprehending that your battle is first won in your heart before it is attained on the battlefield. If discouragement is the loss of courage hope, and heart, then what we need is a dose of encouragement. In contrast, encouragement is often filled with courage, hope, and strength. In Haggai 2:4–5 the scripture states, "Yet now **be strong**, O Zerubbabel, saith the LORD; and **be strong**, O Joshua, son of Josedech, the high priest; and **be strong**, all ye people of the land, saith the LORD, and work: for I am with you, saith the LORD of hosts: According to the word that I covenanted with you when ye came out of Egypt, so my spirit remaineth among you: fear ye not." Three times the Lord tells his people, **"Be strong!"** God is letting us know through this story that when you face life's challenges you must realize the battle is first won in your heart before it is attained on the battlefield of life.

The story of THE THREE TREES helps to shed more light on this issue of wanting to quit. However, we will discover also that trusting in the promises of God always brings unique results.

Once there were three trees on a hill in the woods. They were discussing their hopes and dreams when the first tree said,

"Someday I hope to be a treasure chest. I could be filled with gold, silver, and precious gems. I could be decorated with intricate carving and everyone would see the beauty."

Then the second tree said, "Someday I will be a mighty ship. I will take kings and queens across the waters and sail to the corners of the world. Everyone will feel safe in me because of the strength of my hull."

Finally, the third tree said, "I want to grow to be the tallest and straightest tree in the forest. People will see me on top of the hill and look up to my branches, and think of the heavens and God and how close to them I am reaching. I will be the greatest tree of all time and people will always remember me."

After a few years of praying that their dreams would come true, a group of woodsmen came upon the trees.

One woodsman came to the first tree, "This looks like a strong tree, and I think I should be able to sell the wood to a carpenter." Thus, he began cutting it down. The tree was happy, because he knew that the carpenter would make him into a treasure chest.

At the second tree a woodsman said, "This looks like a strong tree, I should be able to sell it to the shipyard." The second tree was happy because he knew he was on his way to becoming a mighty ship.

When the woodsman came upon the third tree, the tree was frightened because he knew that if they cut him down his dreams would not come true. One of the woodsmen said, "I do not need anything special from my tree so I'll take this one," and he cut it down.

When the first tree arrived at the carpenters, he was made into a feed box for animals. He was then placed in a barn and filled with hay. This was not at all, what he had prayed.

The second tree was cut and made into a small fishing boat. His dreams of being a mighty ship and carrying kings had come to an end.

The third tree was cut into large pieces and left alone in the dark. The years went by, and the trees forgot about their dreams.

One day, a man and woman came to the barn. She gave birth and they placed the baby in the hay in the feed box that was made from the first tree. The man wished that he could have made a crib for the baby, but this manger would have to do.

> QUITTING TOO SOON CAN SPOIL THE MIRACLE

The FIRST tree could feel the importance of this event and knew that it had held the greatest treasure of all time.

Years later, a group of men got in the fishing boat made from the second tree. One of them was tired and went to sleep. While they were out on the water, a great storm arose and the tree did not think it was strong enough to keep the men safe. The men woke the sleeping man, and he stood and said "Peace" and the storm stopped.

At that very moment, the SECOND tree knew that it had carried the King of Kings in its boat.

Finally, someone came and got the THIRD tree. It was carried through the streets as the people mocked the man who was carrying it. When they came to a stop, the man was nailed to the tree and raised in the air to die at the top of a hill. When Sunday morning came, the tree realized Jesus died on that tree but rose from the dead!

In short, when things do not seem to be going according to your plans, always know that God has a wonderful plan for you.

Each of the trees got what they wanted, just not in the way they had imagined!!

When thoughts of quitting enter my mind, I hum the old gospel song, *I Don't Feel No Ways Tired* by Dr. James Cleveland. A portion of the words to this song is as follows: "I don't feel no ways tired, come too far from where I started. Nobody told me that the road would be easy—I don't believe He brought me this far to leave me!"

We may not know exactly what God has planned for our lives. Be assured that you will not want to miss it, and we will never know what His best was if we quit. Jeremiah 29:11 declares, "For I know the thoughts that I think toward you, saith the LORD, thoughts of peace, and not of evil, to give you an expected end." In short, God will pull you through if you can stand the pull.

Wanting to quit, I have been there. I second that emotion!

SMALL GROUP DISCUSSION QUESTIONS:

1. List five instances that made you entertain the thought of wanting to quit.

2. Write a short sentence prayer to God that expresses your reasons for wanting to quit.

3. What strategies did you employ to help you deal with your desire to quit? Do you believe that you utilized healthy strategies? Please explain.

4. Do you believe that everyone in the world has thought about quitting? Why or why not?

5. Did the author provide you with some motivational tips to help you to continue to achieve your dreams and goals while in the midst of obvious opposition? Please explain.

Book
Reviews and
Endorsements

I *Second That Emotion* by Pastor Darron Edwards is a well-written, informative book on seven human emotions that influence the lifestyle of church and individual both positively and negatively. However, this book is quick to give Biblical and Christ-like solutions either to overcome those emotions or to harness them for the glory of God. Pastor Edwards' humanity shows through in a positive way to reveal to the reader that they too can be victorious in the emotional arena.

—Dr. Nodell Dennis, National President, Southern Baptist Conference of Associational Directors of Missions Executive Director, Blue River-Kansas City Baptist Association

Darron Edwards captures the moment with his sharp focus on seven emotions that affect us all. Pastor Edwards skillfully leads us through a deliverance journey that will indeed enlighten and provide positive steps to conquer what is holding us hostage.

When you reach the last page, you will say thank you Pastor Edwards for allowing me to rediscover the joy, peace, and the desire to hold on and hold out. You will once again discover the laughter from within that for so long has been on an emotional vacation. As you read this work, you will need to "buckle up and enjoy the journey."

—**Dr. Donald D. Ford, I, Pastor/Founder Second Missionary Baptist Church of Grandview, Missouri Chancellor, Joel Ecclesiastical School of Preparation**

With a subject matter that is universally relevant but many times unfortunately repressed, Pastor Darron Edwards, with crystal-clear analogies and linguistic giftedness, brings the issues of life up off the written pages to become 'living epistles' in our own hearts. *I Second That Emotion* is second to none, in meeting us right were we are and speaking to us just what we need. Now, I Second That Emotion.

—**A. Louis Patterson, III Pastor/Founder "The L.O.V.E" Church of Dallas, Texas**

This God-breathed work is a most helpful book providing insightful information on emotions. Darron Edwards walks the reader through these often experienced, yet seldom dealt with, emotions that affect our worship life, our work life, and our wedded life. He offers practical application and biblical principles to help the reader deal with them in the right way. *I Second That Emotion* offers real hope and the promise of victory in Jesus to those battling with their emotions. It is an essential tool for church leaders, families, and friends desiring to help those whose emotions seem to be getting the best of them.

—Douglas E. Brown, Pastor/Teacher
Great Commission Baptist
Church of Fort
Worth, Texas

I want to thank my friend and brother, Pastor Darron Edwards for asking me to review his book, *I Second That Emotion*. Pastor Edwards meant it for one thing, but God used it to accomplish much more. For in my reading to write a review God used this book to revive my own spirit. Once I started reading, I could not put it down until I finished. *I Second That Emotion* is a must read book for every Pastor and Laymen who has ever had any thoughts of quitting. Thank you Pastor Edwards for listening to the words of Pastor Ralph D. West, "You have a great gift of writing."

—Dr. Jerry William Dailey,
Pastor Macedonia Baptist
Church of San
Antonio, Texas

I find the godly insights of Pastor Darron Edwards both exciting and refreshing at a time when the Body of Christ is faced with ever challenging nuisances. The "seven plagues," as depicted in this book, are no strangers to the Body of Christ, yet God provides a way to deal with these menaces for the believer. The author's practical and biblical approach is a "must read" for ministries all over the country intent on helping people to heal the hurting soul.

—State Overseer Kenneth B. Spears
First Saint John Full Gospel Baptist
Church, Fort Worth, Texas

There are issues that affect pulpit and pew that are rarely discussed and it is a greater rarity to have a resource that you can direct a colleague, member, or even use for yourself. Rev. Darron Edwards has been divinely led to deal with these issues in a format that is understandable and provokes questions. *I Second That Emotion* will take the reader on a self-examination of emotions of anger, depression, grief, guilt, loneliness, stress and wanting to give up that go beyond a simple topical solution, but seeks to take the reader through practical, thorough and most of all, Biblical solutions. It is a must-have for all progressively minded pastors and laypersons.

—Dr. Robert E. Houston, Sr., Pastor
New Hope Friendship Baptist
Church of San
Diego, California

What a wonderfully inspiring book! Pastor Edwards has a way of putting difficult issues into perspective, making life's problems easier to identify, as well as confront in a positive, pro-active manner. As Pastor Edwards shows us throughout the book, with God, all things are possible. When it comes to living a healthier, more productive life, *I Second That Emotion* provides a wealth of goodly and Godly direction. Whether you are hurting, healing, or helping, Pastor Edwards' book is a great resource."

—Mr. Neal White
Publisher/Editor of the
Waxahachie Daily Light
of Waxahachie, Texas

We have all been given the ability to respond to life's situations naturally as well as spiritually. In the natural, life can be challenging especially when our emotions run together, become unmanageable, and seemingly get the best of us. Pastor

Darron Edwards in this literature gives us counsel on how not to allow our emotions to run rampant. Thus, things in our natural experience begin to dictate our spiritual life. Every one will sense pain, hurt, anger, frustration, love, guilt, and depression, but the question is what you should do with it! After reading this book, I am sure you will be changed forever—Bless you *Edwards!*

—**Marc L. Neal, Pastor Jerusalem Baptist Church of Akron, Ohio**

To order additional copies of

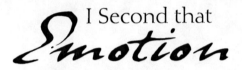 I Second that
Emotion

Have your credit card ready and call:

1-877-421-READ (7323)

or please visit our web site at
www.pleasantword.com

Also available at:
www.amazon.com
and
www.barnesandnoble.com

Printed in the United States
65434LVS00002B/34-48